Antisocial Personality Disorder

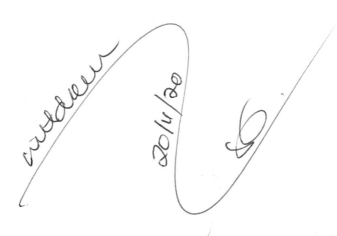

PAUL MORAN

Antisocial Personality Disorder

An Epidemiological Perspective

GASKELL

Gaskell is an imprint of the Royal College of Psychiatrists,
17 Belgrave Square, London SW1X 8PG

British Library Cataloguing-in-Publication Data
A catalogue record for this book is available from
the British Library.
ISBN 0-901242-24-2

Distributed in North America
by American Psychiatric Press, Inc.
ISBN 0-88048-594-9

Printed by Henry Ling Limited, Dorchester, Dorset

Contents

Acknowledgements   vi

Introduction   viii

1   Introduction to the epidemiological review   1
2   Descriptive studies   10
3   Natural history studies   43
4   Studies of associated conditions   55
5   Studies of risk factors   70
6   Social and health care burden of antisocial personality disorder   85
7   Needs assessment   91
8   Conclusions and recommendations   100

References   104

Index   121

Acknowledgements

This book is based on a review that was commissioned and funded by the High Security Psychiatric Services Commissioning Board. I would like to thank the Board and particularly Dr Dilys Jones for providing me with the opportunity to undertake this research. My interest in personality disorder was initially stimulated by experience gained while working on Professor Mann's unit at the Maudsley Hospital. I am indebted to him for his guidance and encouragement throughout my training in psychiatry. My supervisors, Dr Rachel Jenkins and Professor Mann, provided unstinting advice and support throughout the project, and I would like to thank them for this. I am grateful to Professor Jeremy Coid, Professor John Gunn and Professor Pamela Taylor, who drew my attention to valuable references in the literature of forensic psychiatry. Professor Gunn and Professor Taylor also kindly made helpful comments on the draft of the initial review.

The following individuals provided me with information, advice and encouragement: Dr Sube Banerjee (Institute of Psychiatry, London), Dr Jonathan Bindman (Institute of Psychiatry, London), Professor Nick Black (London School of Hygiene and Tropical Medicine), Professor Tony Culyer (Department of Economics and Related Studies, University of York), Professor Conor Duggan (Department of Forensic Psychiatry, University of Leicester), Professor David Farrington (Institute of Criminology, Cambridge), Dr Robert Goodman (Institute of Psychiatry, London), Dr Gisli Gudjonsson (Institute of Psychiatry, London), Dr Mari Harty (Broadmoor Hospital, Berkshire), Dr Ian Keitch (Rampton Hospital, Nottingham), Sylvia Kingaby (Department of Health, London), Dr Leo Kroll (Cherry Tree Hospital, Stockport), Dr Emmet Larkin (Rampton Hospital, Nottingham), Dr Anthony Maden (Institute of Psychiatry, London), Dr Howard Meltzer (Office of National Statistics, London), Professor Marshall Marinker (High Security Psychiatric Services Commissioning Board, London), James Potts

(Department of Health, London), Mike Preston (High Security Psychiatric Services Commissioning Board, London), Professor Graham Thornicroft (Institute of Psychiatry, London).

Finally, I would like to thank my father, Dr Emanuel Moran, whose clarity of thought and determination of spirit has always been a great source of inspiration to me.

Paul Moran
Section of Epidemiology and General Practice
Institute of Psychiatry
London
July 1998

Introduction

It has been suggested that the personality disorders "constitute one of the most important sources of long-term impairment in treated and untreated populations" (Merikangas & Weissman, 1986). Arguably, from the perspective of health and social service planners and the criminal justice system, the group posing one of the greatest challenges is of those with personality disorder who offend. Recognition of the importance of this group to the National Health Service is provided by the fact that in the 1994/95 priorities and planning guidance for the NHS, services for mentally disordered offenders, including people with antisocial and psychopathic personality disorders, are a "first order priority". Nevertheless, the importance of personality disorders as a source of social cost and burden, and patient morbidity and mortality, is often under-appreciated (Oldham, 1994). The High Security Psychiatric Services Commissioning Board commissioned this review at a time of a resurgence of interest into personality disorders in order to help underpin a new portfolio of research in this area.

Recently, there have been several important initiatives concerning the management of psychopathic disorder which include the Reed Report (Department of Health & Home Office, 1994) with its accompanying literature review by Dolan & Coid (1993) and the recent contentious introduction of Hybrid Orders, by the Crime (Sentences) Act 1997 for individuals suffering from psychopathic disorder (Eastman & Peay, 1998). This book, therefore, appears at a time of enhanced activity, and it is hoped that it will provide a balanced epidemiological perspective on a difficult subject; one which continues to attract controversy and debate.

Aims of the review

Ultimately, the aim of this book is to inform the reader on the current state of knowledge about the frequency, distribution, natural history and associated burden of antisocial personality disorder and its diagnostic equivalents: dissocial personality disorder, sociopathy and psychopathy. It should be emphasised that the European medical profession has largely given up the term 'psychopathy'. Moreover, the process of literature-searching revealed only a very slim collection of epidemiological studies concerning psychopathy. For these reasons, for the most part, the review concerns itself largely with the epidemiology of antisocial personality disorder. Epidemiologists are increasingly preoccupied with the assessment of need, and in the light of this, a chapter has been included on this subject as it relates to antisocial personality disorder.

It was not my intention to produce a detailed analysis of the concept of psychopathy, nor a lengthy discussion of its chequered history. These aspects have been extensively and eloquently covered by a number of luminaries from the fields of psychiatry and psychology, and to add to them would seem to be a rather fruitless exercise. What does, however, seem to have been missing is a synthesis and evaluation of the large amount of published epidemiological research into antisocial personality disorder and psychopathy. This book is intended to fill that gap.

Methodology

Literature-searching is a vital component of any systematic review (University of York, 1996). A number of sources of material were used to facilitate the literature-searching process. First, a computerised database search of relevant publications in scientific journals covering the past three decades was conducted using CD-ROM Medline and PsychLit. This list of publications was supplemented by handsearching key scientific journals to identify articles which were missed in the database search. Handsearched journals included *Criminal Behaviour and Mental Health*, the *British Journal of Forensic Psychiatry* and the *British Journal of Criminology*. In addition, Department of Health and special hospitals data concerning admission rates were collated and are included in the review. Second, a number of researchers and clinicians with an interest in the fields of epidemiology and forensic psychiatry were identified and invited to provide information about any recent or unpublished work – a list of these contributors is included in the Acknowledgements of this book.

Where possible, findings have been tabulated, and where data of a reasonably high quality were identified, the findings have been synthesised to form a consensus view. Methodological issues with respect to the assessment of the epidemiological characteristics of antisocial personality disorder have been discussed. The review concludes by offering some suggestions for future research in the light of these issues.

One of the aims of the book is to provide as comprehensive a list as possible of published and unpublished epidemiological studies of antisocial personality disorder and its diagnostic equivalents. The following points should, however, be noted. First, only two databases were used in the literature search. Second, databases do not record all publications from all medical journals (Dickersin *et al*, 1994). Third, the review only sampled studies written in English. Thus, like all reviews, there is the danger that some relevant studies will have been inadvertently missed in the process of gathering pertinent literature. The author regrets any omissions.

The concept of psychopathy and its relationship to antisocial personality disorder

The concepts of antisocial personality disorder and psychopathy are closely linked, the former representing an attempt to operationalise the latter older term. For this important reason, before turning to the epidemiological literature, it is necessary to consider the nature of this relationship.

As Lewis (1974) has noted, "psychopathic personality" is one of a group of terms to have been used over the past 150 years in order to denote abnormal personality. Other "semantic variations on a dubious theme" have included moral insanity, moral imbecility and constitutional immorality. Up until the late 19th century the adjective 'psychopathic' meant 'psychopathological' and applied to any form of mental disorder (Berrios, 1993). Koch (1891), however, introduced the plural form "psychopathic inferiorities", in order to refer to a group of abnormal behavioural states which fell midway between mental disorder and normality. The underlying aetiology was presumed to be a physical one and a range of disturbance was proposed to occur, which included severely antisocial behaviour. Kraepelin (1899) used the term "psychopathic personalities" in a more general sense to mean degenerative disorders of the personality, although Schneider (1950) later refined the meaning of the term to refer to a subclass of the abnormal personalities who "suffer, or make society suffer, on account of their abnormality". This subclass consisted of 10 variants of psychopathological personality and formed the foundation of the present international classifications. More recently, the term psychopathy has disappeared from contemporary classifications, although its essence has survived in the

Diagnostic and Statistical Manual of Mental Disorders (DSM–IV; American Psychiatric Association, 1994) category of antisocial personality disorder and in the International Classification of Diseases (ICD–10; World Health Organization, 1992) as dissocial personality disorder.

Over the past 70 years, an extensive literature on the subject of psychopathy has been generated, much of which is, in the words of Aubrey Lewis (1974), "disheartening...... (and characterised by) fine-spun theorising, repetitive argument and therapeutic gloom". Strong arguments have been made for abandoning the term on the grounds that it is a pejorative label which does not refer to a single category of identifiable individuals (Walker & McCabe, 1973; Home Office & Department of Health and Social Security, 1975; Gunn & Robertson, 1976; Blackburn, 1988). However, in spite of intense criticism, the term has survived and, to quote Dolan & Coid (1993), "outlived its obituarists". Moreover, in North America, largely due to the work of Robert Hare, psychopathy has recently undergone something of a renaissance, with a large amount of research being generated to support Hare's conceptualisation of the disorder.

Currently, the term psychopathy has three uses: as a clinical construct (although one which is now rarely used in the UK); as a legal category of mental disorder under the English Mental Health Act 1983 (in the guise of psychopathic disorder); and in the vernacular as a term of derogation.

In legal terms, the Mental Health Act 1983 defines psychopathic disorder as: "A persistent disorder or disability of mind (whether or not including significant impairment of intelligence) which results in abnormally aggressive or seriously irresponsible conduct."

Used in this context, psychopathic disorder is one of four specific categories of 'mental disorder' through which a patient may be compulsorily admitted to hospital. The 'elastic' and vague interpretation of this legal category has led to its severe criticism (Chiswick, 1992). In addition, research indicates that many 'legally-defined psychopaths' are not in fact 'clinical psychopaths' as defined by an instrument such as the Psychopathy Checklist (Coid, 1992). Because of these concerns, the category is now used comparatively rarely as a means of achieving the compulsory admission of a patient to hospital. Between 1990/91 and 1995/96 there were only 101 formal admissions to psychiatric hospital under the legal category of psychopathic disorder. This contrasts with 144 for mental impairment and 10 099 for mental illness (Department of Health, 1997).

Although now rarely used in this country, the clinical construct has recently been revived in North America. In their review of psychopathy written over 50 years ago, Curran & Mallinson (1944) concluded that research into the subject could not be taken any further until "more agreement has been reached on questions of definition and delimitation". When reading contemporary literature on the subject, one experiences a sense of *déjà vu*, since although studies of the clinical construct of psychopathy are once again proliferating, there remains a fundamental disagreement concerning the best way to conceptualise this construct (Davies & Feldman, 1981; Lilienfeld, 1994). Whereas some authors believe that psychopathy should be conceptualised principally in terms of personality traits, others believe that it is better viewed in terms of antisocial behaviour.

The most influential proponent of the personality-based approach has been Cleckley (1941), who in his book *The Mask of Sanity* delineated 16 criteria for the diagnosis of psychopathy. These criteria included superficial charm, lack of anxiety, lack of guilt, undependability, dishonesty, egocentricity, failure to form lasting intimate relationships, failure to learn from punishment, poverty of emotions, lack of insight into the impact of one's behaviour upon others, and failure to plan ahead. Hare (1980) has taken these characteristics, applied them to a series of prisoners and developed the Psychopathy Checklist (PCL). Hare and his colleagues argue that psychopathy is a unitary syndrome that can be measured using the PCL. A series of studies has led to the development of a revised (20-item) Psychopathy Checklist (PCL–R; Hare, 1991), and the psychometric properties of this instrument and its clinical utility in predicting violent offending and recidivism are well documented (e.g. Harris *et al*, 1991; Hart & Hare, 1994). The items in the revised Psychopathy Checklist are summarised in Table 1. Two factors have been shown to be measured by different subsets of items in the PCL–R. Factor 1 consists of items that describe a cluster of affective–interpersonal traits central to the classical description of the psychopath. Factor 2 comprises items that describe traits and behaviours associated with an unstable and antisocial lifestyle.

Although the Cleckley/Hare model of psychopathy has received a great deal of enthusiastic support (largely in North America), it is not without its critics. The model seems to be uncomfortably close to a moral concept, and for some critics represents a disguised attempt to study the concept of evil scientifically (J. Gunn, personal communication, 1997). In a similar vein, the scientific validity of an instrument that measures common moral attitudes such as 'parasitic' or 'irresponsible' should be questioned. Others have highlighted the irony of Hare's claim that the DSM–IV antisocial personality disorder criteria are too crime-centred, while at the same time demonstrating the 'superiority' of the PCL–R over the DSM criteria by finding that the PCL–R is a better predictor of criminal recidivism (Robins, 1995).

TABLE 1
Summary of items in the revised (20-item) Psychopathy Checklist (PCL–R)

1. Glibness/superficial charm	11. Promiscuous sexual behaviour
2. Grandiose sense of self-worth	12. Early behavioural problems
3. Need for stimulation/ proneness to boredom	13. Lack of realistic, long-term goals
4. Pathological lying	14. Impulsivity
5. Cunning/manipulative	15. Irresponsibility
6. Lack of remorse or guilt	16. Failure to accept responsibility for own actions
7. Shallow affect	17. Many short-term marital relationships
8. Callous/lack of empathy	18. Juvenile delinquency
9. Parasitic lifestyle	19. Revocation of conditional release
10. Poor behavioural controls	20. Criminal versatility

Proponents of the behaviour-based approach to the conceptuali-sation of psychopathy argue that the personality approach requires too much inference, and is likely to possess low interrater reliability (Cloninger, 1978; Robins, 1978). It is argued that observation of behaviour is likely to be a more reliable process. Within this scheme, antisocial behaviour is the cornerstone for the diagnosis of psycho-pathy, and psychopathy is equated with a diagnosis of antisocial personality disorder in DSM–IV and dissocial personality disorder in ICD–10. The diagnostic criteria for each of these categories are given in Tables 2 and 3. In contrast to DSM–III–R, the DSM–IV criteria are much closer to those of ICD–10, a feature which is in keeping with the growing comparability of the two classificatory systems (Sara *et al*, 1996). The ICD–10 criteria emphasise personality characteristics, and as such have been commended for presenting a more complete diagnostic picture of psychopathy, although data concerning their reliability or validity have yet to be published.

DSM–IV antisocial personality disorder has previously been described as "the most controversial of all the personality disorders" (Frances, 1980). Certainly the diagnosis merits such a description purely on the basis of the substantial criticism which it has received. Much of this criticism is aimed at the fact that there is an overemphasis on overt criminal acts and related behaviours, and a neglect of the more general Cleckleyan personality traits of psychopathy. Widiger & Corbitt (1995) have suggested that this has contributed to:

(a) a failure to represent traditional concepts of psychopathy adequately;

TABLE 2

Summary of the DSM–IV diagnostic criteria for antisocial personality disorder

---

A. Pervasive pattern of disregard for and violation of rights of others, occurring since age 15 years, as indicated by 3 (or more) of the following:
   (1) failure to conform to social norms with respect to lawful behaviours
   (2) deceitfulness
   (3) impulsivity
   (4) irritability and aggressiveness
   (5) reckless disregard for safety of self or others
   (6) consistent irresponsibility
   (7) lack of remorse
B. Current age at least 18 years
C. Evidence of conduct disorder with onset before 15 years
D. Occurrence of antisocial behaviour is not exclusively during the course of schizophrenia or a manic episode

---

Reprinted with permission from DSM–IV (copyright American Psychiatric Association, 1994).

(b) an overdiagnosis of antisocial personality disorder in criminal settings (termed "the over-inclusiveness problem") and the suggestion by some that "criminality and sociopathic personality are overlapping terms – if not entirely synonymous" (Guze *et al*, 1967);

(c) an underdiagnosis of antisocial personality disorder in non-criminal settings (termed "the under-inclusiveness problem");

(d) difficulties in the differentiation of antisocial personality disorder from substance use disorders; and

(e) an overly complex and cumbersome criteria set.

Despite these major criticisms, antisocial personality disorder is the only personality disorder diagnosis that consistently demonstrates adequate to good levels of interrater reliability in routine practice (Mellsop *et al*, 1982), and adequate to good convergent validity with semi-structured interview and self-report assessments (Skodol *et al*, 1991). It is also the only category of personality disorder to have been consistently studied in the major community-based epidemiological surveys. In addition, the DSM criteria represent the only personality disorder category that is derived from empirical research. (The criteria directly originate from Lee Robins' 30-year follow-up study of children referred to a child guidance clinic (Robins, 1966, 1978), the main findings of which are summarised on pp. 44–45.)

The DSM–IV field trial (Widiger *et al*, 1996) attempted to answer some of the questions raised by the behaviour/trait debate by comparing the validity, reliability and correlation with external validators of DSM–III–R antisocial personality disorder criteria, ICD–10 dissocial personality disorder criteria, and PCL–R-derived criteria.

TABLE 3
Summary of the diagnostic criteria for ICD–10 dissocial personality disorder

(a) Callous unconcern for the feelings of others
(b) Gross and persistent attitude of irresponsibility and disregard for social norms, rules and obligations
(c) Incapacity to maintain enduring relationships, though having no difficulty in establishing them
(d) Very low tolerance to frustration and a low threshold for discharge of aggression, including violence
(e) Incapacity to experience guilt and to profit from experience, particularly punishment
(f) Marked proneness to blame others, or to offer plausible rationalisations, for the behaviour that has brought the patient into conflict with society

Reprinted with permission from ICD–10 (copyright World Health Organization, 1992).

The current DSM–IV criteria for antisocial personality disorder (American Psychiatric Association, 1994) represent an attempt to incorporate the revisions suggested by the trial and are summarised in Table 2. The field trial has, however, been heavily criticised for failing to address adequately the problems of reliability and content-related validity (Hare & Hart, 1995). In the light of these criticisms, it is difficult to be sure whether or not the DSM–IV criteria represent an advance in the conceptualisation of the clinical construct of psychopathy.

In summary, psychiatry has demonstrated an inability to rid itself of the term psychopathy. Although abandoned from current classification schemes, its spirit lives on in the guise of antisocial personality disorder (a disorder which, as this book will demonstrate, has generated a large literature and, by doing so, taken on a life of its own). Enthusiasm for the revival of the clinical construct of psychopathy is largely based in North America, where the PCL–R is becoming an increasingly integral part of forensic psychiatric practice (Cooke, 1997). However, even if we accept the notion of a unitary clinical construct termed psychopathy, there exists no agreement within psychiatry as to how this construct should best be conceptualised. Almost 25 years have now elapsed since Aubrey Lewis published his famous critique on the subject, yet with regard to psychopathy the only issue upon which psychiatrists are agreed is that the concept remains 'most elusive'.

Studies included in the review

Psychopathy's elusiveness has considerable ramifications for the consideration of epidemiological 'caseness', and complicates the selection of studies for inclusion in an epidemiological review.

Although this book is primarily concerned with antisocial personality disorder, in the light of the aforementioned historical links with psychopathy, where relevant, epidemiological studies of psychopathy have been included. For similar reasons, studies of sociopathy and of dissocial personality disorder have also been included. Given the evidence of multiple morbidity of personality disorder diagnoses in subjects with severe personality disorder (e.g. Dolan *et al*, 1995), the increasing evidence for diagnostic overlap between antisocial personality disorder and borderline personality disorder (e.g. Paris, 1997*b*), and evidence that there has been a tendency to diagnose borderline personality disorder in those who would previously have been diagnosed as suffering from psychopathy (Simonsen & Mellergard, 1988), a case could also have been made for including epidemiological studies of borderline personality disorder. This was, however, considered to be beyond the scope of this review. Pure studies of the epidemiology of crime were also considered to be beyond the scope of this review, although where they relate directly to antisocial personality (such as in the area of risk factors) they were included. The author acknowledges that given the emphasis that current operationalised criteria place on behavioural characteristics of antisocial personality disorder, a case could have been made for the inclusion of such studies.

Two further areas are notable in their omission from the review. There is a growing literature on the neurobiological correlates of psychopathy. It is the author's belief that a comprehensive review of this important area is beyond the scope of a book whose primary aim is to deal with central epidemiological issues. A recent review of the literature on the biology of psychopathy concluded that "from a biological perspective, the literature on aetiological factors in psychopathy is confusing and inconsistent, largely because of variations in diagnostic criteria" (Dolan, 1994). Presumably mindful of this, recent biological research has attempted to use more clearly defined subjects (e.g. Kuruoglu *et al*, 1996; Intrator *et al*, 1997), although presently, clear biological markers of antisocial personality disorder and psychopathy have yet to be identified. Finally, studies of the treatment of psychopathic and antisocial personality disorders have been recently and comprehensively reviewed by Dolan & Coid (1993), and in order to avoid unnecessary duplication, this area has also been omitted.

1 Introduction to the epidemiological review

The word epidemiology is a term used in medicine to designate the study of populations rather than individuals. More specifically, and from a narrowly defined perspective, epidemiology is concerned with the distribution of diseases in a population and the factors that influence that distribution (Lilienfield, 1957). A broader definition extends the value of epidemiology to incorporate studies that test aetiological hypotheses and which examine factors that influence course and outcome. Morris (1957) summarised the 'uses' of epidemiology as follows: (a) community diagnosis; (b) completion of the clinical picture of disease; (c) delineation of new syndromes; (d) computation of individual morbid risk; (e) charting historical trends; (f) evaluation of health services; and (g) identification of causal factors.

For the purpose of this review, a broader definition of epidemiology has been adopted. The reviewed studies fall into one of the following five categories:

Descriptive studies

Under this category are included all studies that provide information about the distribution and frequency of antisocial personality disorder and its diagnostic equivalents in a variety of populations. The majority of the literature reviewed fell into this category. Four population settings were looked at: the community, primary care, secondary care and other institutions (prisons and special hospitals).

Natural history studies

These include studies that examine levels of recovery and disability at follow-up.

1

Studies of associated conditions

These include studies of associated axis I and axis II conditions.

Risk factor studies

These include prospective and retrospective studies (usually adopting a case–control design) of deviant/high-risk children and adults with antisocial personality disorder.

Studies of the cost and burden associated with psychopathy

These include studies of societal costs in terms of indices such as family violence, unemployment, crime and heavy health service utilisation.

In epidemiological studies of axis I disorders, such as depression and schizophrenia, there is comparatively little disagreement about who to interview, when to interview, or even what measure to use (Zimmerman, 1994). Unfortunately, life is not so simple for the worker conducting personality disorder research. Before the main findings of the review are presented, it is important to put them in the context of the considerable challenges involved in classifying and assessing personality disorders generally.

Problems in the assessment of personality disorders

By their very nature, personality disorders present a multitude of measurement problems. First, unlike axis I disorders, they are diagnosed in an interpersonal context and are nearly totally dependent upon the assessment of characteristic patterns of social interaction. Taking the example of DSM–IV antisocial personality disorder, as can be seen from Table 2 in the Introduction, the diagnosis requires, among other features, evidence of "disregard and violation of the rights of others". Unlike axis I disorders, where an individual's own baseline can be used to generate estimates of the degree of abnormality, the same is not true for personality disorders.

Second, there is good evidence that while personality disorders are, by definition, enduring, they fluctuate considerably with the presence of axis I disorder (e.g. Tyrer, 1987; Mavissakalian, 1990). Some axis I conditions may lead to a personality disorder diagnosis where none in fact exists, and as an example of this Gunderson & Phillips (1994) have cited the hypomanic patient who appears histrionic or narcissistic. It is therefore clear that careful attention should be paid to the subject's current symptomatic state, and re-interviews during a period of remission from axis I disorder may be necessary for an accurate assessment. All of this lengthens the diagnostic assessment and adds to the cost of an epidemiological survey in terms of both time and money.

Third, there are many potential biases that threaten to contaminate the diagnostic impression. Most prominent among these are gender biases and sociocultural biases. It has been suggested that histrionic and dependent personality disorders may represent exaggerated variants of stereotypically feminine behaviour, and thus may be overdiagnosed in women (Gunderson & Phillips, 1994). Similarly, clinicians should be cautious before diagnosing personality disorders in patients from sociocultural backgrounds different to their own. The work of the World Health Organization Alcohol, Drug Abuse and Mental Health Administration programme has, however, demonstrated that it is possible to assess personality disorder in different nations, languages and cultures using a semi-structured interview, the International Personality Disorder Examination (Loranger *et al*, 1994).

Fourth, because of the recency of interest in personality disorders, there is less experience in assessing them and fewer instruments available for this purpose. Essentially, three methods are available for the assessment of personality disorders: unstandardised clinical interviews, standardised clinical interviews (usually semi-structured) and self-report questionnaires. Some of the main instruments for assessing all personality disorders are shown in Table 1.1. The following general points can be stated in relation to the psychometric properties of the available instruments:

(a) The interrater reliability of the majority of instruments is good although, as Zimmerman (1994) concluded in his review of the area, this may only hold for when the instruments are used by their developers.

(b) The test–retest reliability of the majority of instruments is poorer, although the Personality Assessment Schedule (PAS; Tyrer *et al*, 1979), the International Personality Disorder Examination (IPDE; Loranger *et al*, 1994) and the Standardised Assessment of Personality (SAP; Pilgrim & Mann, 1990) yield diagnoses with more satisfactory temporal stability.

(c) It is now generally accepted that there is poor agreement between a diagnosis of personality disorder obtained by self-report questionnaire and that obtained by a clinical interview (Hyler *et al*, 1989). In addition, poor concordance has been found to exist between standardised interviews and self-report questionnaires. Perry (1992) reviewed the concordance

TABLE 1.1
Assessment methods for all personality disorders (adapted from De Girolamo & Reich (1993) courtesy of the World Health Organization)

Instrument	Author	Method	Number of items	Time required (min)
Diagnostic Interview for Personality Disorders (DIPD)	Zanarini (1983)	Semi-structured interview with patient using DSM–III–R criteria	101	60–120
International Personality Disorder Examination (IPDE)	Loranger et al (1991)	Semi-structured interview with patient using ICD–10 and DSM–III–R criteria	157	150
Millon Clinical Multiaxial Inventory (MCMI)	Millon (1982)	Self-report by patient using DSM–III–R criteria	175	20–30
Personality Assessment Schedule (PAS)	Tyrer et al (1979)	Semi-structured interview with informant(s) using DSM–III–R criteria	24	60
Personality Diagnostic Questionnaire - Revised (PDQ–R)	Hyler & Reider (1984)	Self-report by patient or informant(s) using DSM–III–R criteria	152	30
Personality Interview Questions II (PIQ–II)	Widiger (1987)	Semi-structured interview with patient using DSM–III criteria	106	60–120

contd....

TABLE 1.1 (*contd...*)

Schedule for Normal & Abnormal Personality Disorders (SNAP)	Clark (1989)	Self-report by patient using DSM–III and dimensional criteria	375	10
Standardised Assessment of Personality (SAP)	Pilgrim & Mann (1990)	Semi-structured interview with informant(s) using ICD–10 and DSM–III–R criteria	NA	10–15
Structured Clinical Interview for DSM–III–R Personality Disorders (SCID–II)	Spitzer & Williams (1987)	Semi-structured interview with patient using DSM–III–R criteria	120	60–90
Structured Interview for DSM–III Personality Disorders (SIPD)	Pfohl *et al* (1983)	Semi-structured interview with patient or informant(s) using DSM–III criteria	136	90
Tridimensional Personality Questionnaire (TPQ)	Cloninger (1987)	Self-report by patient	100	20–30
Wisconsin Personality Inventory (WISPI)	Klein (1985)	Self-report by patient using DSM–III criteria	360	20

between standardised interviews and self-report questionnaires for the diagnosis of personality disorders. On the basis of eight studies in which two or more diagnostic methods were used to assess patients for axis II disorder, the overall level of agreement between interview and self-report questionnaire was low (median kappa value = 0.25). (The use of self-report questionnaires for the eliciting of antisocial symptoms has been criticised, since the deceptiveness associated with antisocial personality disorder is likely to lead to significant under-reporting of symptoms. In the light of this, the need for independent verification of information in the diagnostic assessment process is perhaps more important for antisocial personality disorder than for any other category of personality disorder.)

Finally, a major unresolved issue in the assessment of personality disorders is the determination of which source of information is the most valid – patient or informant. To complicate matters further, it is unclear what constitutes a good or bad informant (Brothwell *et al*, 1992). It should be emphasised that the majority of instruments rely on an interview with the subject and, in the light of some of the potential sources of bias discussed above, there are hazards in this approach (Tyrer, 1995).

Problems in the classification of personality disorders

Although the existence of personality pathology has been recognised since the time of the ancient Greeks, the issue of how best to conceptualise this pathology has remained unresolved. Put simply, the conceptual problem is one of whether personality disorders should be considered to exist along dimensions that reflect extreme variants of normal personality, or whether they should be considered to be categories that qualitatively set them apart from normal personality, similar to categories traditionally used in medicine.

Historically, the very process of attempting to classify something as difficult as abnormal personality has led to an over-reliance on simplistic and caricatured portraits of individuals who are considered flawed in some way. This tradition can be traced back to the 'character writings' of Theophrastus in ancient Greece, and has persisted through to the 19th century in the writings of Prichard ('moral insanity') and to this century with Schneider's influential description of 10 pathological personality types. While such descriptions vividly convey the flaws or foibles of a patient, they fail to capture the subtleties and contradictions inherent in human nature. Currently, we persist with a categorical approach in the classification of personality pathology and continue to rely heavily on simplified and prototypical descriptions of disordered personality. (For a detailed review of the historical development of the concept of personality disorder, see Millon & Davis, 1995.)

The third edition of the *Diagnostic and Statistical Manual of Mental Disorders* (DSM–III; American Psychiatric Association, 1980) organised mental disorders into two axes, codifying a distinction between illness and personality made by classical approaches to psychopathology. Whereas much of the current interest in the personality disorders is attributed directly to the establishment of a multiaxial approach to classification, there is growing evidence that personality pathology is better conceptualised dimensionally. This evidence surrounds the distribution of the phenotypic features and disabilities associated with personality disorder, and a growing body of evidence that supports the link between normal and disordered personality.

Studies reporting on the distribution of personality traits consistently support a dimensional model. For example, Livesley *et al* (1992) examined the scores of a combined sample of 274 general population and 158 personality-disordered subjects on 100 scales that measured features of personality disorder. They found no evidence of bimodality or points of rarity. In a similar vein, more direct evidence in favour of the dimensional approach comes from studies based on axis II criteria. For example, Widiger *et al* (1986) found that individuals who met a sub-threshold number of criteria were more like those who met none of the criteria. The considerable overlap between diagnostic criteria sets (Morey, 1988) and the substantial covariation among personality disorder diagnoses (e.g. Dolan *et al*, 1995) provide further epidemiological evidence against the categorical approach.

Studies examining the functional disability associated with a diagnosis of personality disorder indicate that dysfunction is a continuous variable, thus providing further evidence against a dichotomous approach to classification. Using the Global Assessment of Functioning Scale on a mixed population of personality-disordered and non-personality-disordered patients, Nakao *et al* (1992) demonstrated that impairment was continuously distributed.

Research into the structure of normal personality provides further evidence in favour of the dimensional approach, by showing that measures of normal personality are predictive of measures of personality disorder. Factor-analytical studies of the distribution of personality traits in the normal population have attempted to identify the most essential elements of personality structure. The five-factor model (Digman, 1990) is one of the products of this approach, and is the model which is currently attracting the greatest support. According to this model, normal and abnormal personality can be captured by evaluation along five dimensions: neuroticism, extraversion, openness to experience, agreeableness, and conscientiousness. Several studies have examined the relationship between these dimensions and measures of personality disorder. For example, Wiggins & Pincus (1989) showed that the five-factor model scales of a personality inventory were predictive of Minnesota Multiphasic Personality Inventory (MMPI) measures of axis II diagnoses. Such evidence supports a link between normal and disordered personality and favours the dimensional scheme.

Thus, it is clear that a growing body of empirical evidence supports a dimensional conceptualisation of personality pathology. Nevertheless, clinicians have tended to favour the categorical approach, largely because it is simpler to use and lends itself more easily to treatment decisions. On this latter point, it has been suggested that the coding of personality disorders on a separate axis may be used to justify pessimism about outcome and indeed to withhold treatment (Livesley *et al*, 1994).

Blackburn (1971, 1975, 1986) has effectively hybridised the dimensional and categorical approaches in order to develop a model of psychopathy. By applying the MMPI to a variety of forensic populations (a trait approach), Blackburn has demonstrated four profiles of personality type (a categorical formulation). Types 1 and 2 are considered to represent two subgroups of psychopaths, whereas types 3 and 4 are considered to be non-psychopathic individuals.

(a) *Type 1: primary or 4–9 type.* This is considered to be close to Cleckley's concept. Individuals are highly extroverted, non-neurotic and guilt-free. They have a high level of impulsivity and are more violent in terms of previous convictions.

(b) *Type 2: secondary or neurotic.* These individuals are introverted, anxious, prone to depression and have a highly abnormal MMPI profile suggestive of paranoid and psychotic disorder. Typically, their criminal histories show more sex offences than type 1.

(c) *Type 3: controlled.* These individuals tend to show a defensive denial about psychological problems. Typically, they are sociable, slightly extrovert and highly controlled.

(d) *Type 4: inhibited.* These individuals are typically less controlled and more suspicious than type 3. In addition, they display dysthymic characteristics and difficulties in interpersonal relationships.

Based on these MMPI profiles, Blackburn has developed a simpler approach using a 10-scale questionnaire, the Special Hospitals Assessment of Personality and Socialisation (Blackburn, 1986). Despite some evidence in favour of the use of this approach as a valid assessment method for psychopathy (e.g. Blackburn, 1986), clinically there is good reason to doubt the reliability of self-report instruments when used with subjects who are, by definition, deceitful.

2   Descriptive studies

This chapter reviews all identified published epidemiological surveys of antisocial personality disorder and its diagnostic equivalents in the following populations: community, primary care, psychiatric settings, prisons and special hospitals. By definition, personality disorders are chronic in nature and the establishment of a precise time of onset in order to calculate their incidence is very difficult. For these reasons, incidence studies of personality disorders are exceedingly rare, and all of the quoted studies in the following section are prevalence studies. A rare example of a study which examined the incidence of antisocial personality disorder is Newman *et al* (1996), who reported data from the Dunedin Multidisciplinary Health and Development Study. This is a longitudinal study of a large (base sample = 1037) unselected birth cohort. The cohort has been assessed with a battery of psychological, medical and sociological measures at ages 3, 5, 7, 9, 11, 13, 15, 18 and 21 years, and provides a unique opportunity to study the prevalence and incidence, natural history and risk factors of a number of mental disorders. Using the Diagnostic Interview Schedule (Robins *et al*, 1981; see below for details), it has been possible to assess the proportion of new cases of antisocial personality disorder at a birth cohort age of 21 years. Newman *et al* (1996) estimated that, of the 31 cases of antisocial personality disorder at age 21, 9.7% were new cases at 21, the remainder (90.3%) being cases before age 21.

Community surveys

Goldberg & Huxley (1980) have demonstrated that selection processes operate on the mentally ill that determine which of them will seek care, have their disturbance detected, are treated in primary care, or are referred for psychiatric care. The community survey should, therefore, in theory, yield the most comprehensive picture of the distribution of mental illness free from selection and referral bias (Mann, 1993). It has been suggested that the community survey is perhaps the most significant of all advances in psychiatric epidemiology (Lloyd & Weich, 1997). Nevertheless, such surveys require conceptual clarity, are costly in terms of time and money, and if clumsily carried out may be quite uninformative.

Dohrenwend & Dohrenwend (1982) have reviewed studies of the prevalence of psychiatric disorders, reported between 1950 and 1978 from Western countries. They described first, second and third 'generations' of epidemiological surveys. First-generation studies (pre-Second World War) were characterised by a heavy reliance on case records or informant interviews for case identification. Stromgren (1950) reviewed the literature on the prevalence of psychiatric disorder prior to 1950. Despite methodological short-comings (particularly in terms of the use of non-random sampling techniques and small sample sizes), Stromgren concluded that there was remarkable consistency across 18 of the 60 studies reviewed, and used the summated data to calculate the lifetime risk for various disorders. The computed lifetime risk for psychopathy was 0.53%.

Second-generation studies used structured interviews of community residents and included studies such as the Stirling County Study (Leighton, 1959) and the Midtown Manhattan Study (Langner & Michael, 1963). In their review of 20 studies published between 1950 and 1978, Dohrenwend & Dohrenwend (1982) calculated that the median prevalence for 'personality disorders' was 4.8% . No figures were given for estimates of the prevalence of antisocial personality disorder or psychopathy. In addition, the estimated figure given is imprecise with a wide range (0.1–36%). Merikangas & Weissman (1986) reviewed estimates of the prevalence of antisocial personality disorder published before the introduction of DSM–III. A summary of their findings is presented in Table 2.1.

Third-generation studies represented a major landmark in psychiatric epidemiology and were characterised by the following features:

TABLE 2.1

Prevalence of antisocial personality disorder in community studies prior to DSM–III (adapted from Merikangas & Weissman , 1986, by kind permission of American Psychiatric Press)

Author	Location	Sample size	Prevalence
Stromgren (1950)	Denmark	45 930	0.5%
Bremer (1951)	Norway	1325	9.4%
Essen-Moller (1956)	Sweden	2550	5.6%
Langner & Michael (1963)	United States	1911	1.9%
Leighton (1959)	Canada	1010	2.9%
Helgason (1981)	Iceland	5395	4.0%

(a) use of diagnostic criteria for definition of specific disorders; (b) use of standardised structured interview schedules for symptom assessment; (c) face to face personal interviews; (d) lay interviewers gathering the data; and (e) computerised data management and analyses.

Of all the personality disorders, antisocial personality disorder has been the most consistently studied in third-generation surveys. The prevalence figures for antisocial personality disorder obtained in third-generation surveys are listed in Table 2.2.

TABLE 2.2
Lifetime prevalence of antisocial personality disorder (DSM–III) in community surveys

Author	Location	Sample	Procedure	Lifetime prevalence
Weissman & Myers (1980)	US	511	SADS–L	0.2%
Baron *et al* (1985)	US	376	SIB SADS	0.5%
Bland *et al* (1988*a*)	Canada	3258	DIS	3.7%
Hwu *et al* (1989)	Taiwan	11 004	DIS	0.14%
Reich *et al* (1989)	US	235	PDQ	0.4%
Wells *et al* (1989)	New Zealand	1498	DIS	3.1%
Lee *et al* (1990)	Korea	3134 (urban) 1966 (rural)	DIS	2.1% (urban) 0.9% (rural)
Zimmerman & Coryell (1990)	US	697	PDQ SIDP	0.9% 3.0%
Robins & Regier (1991)	US (ECA)	18 571	DIS	2.4%
Maier *et al* (1992)	Germany	447	SCID–II	0.2%
Chen *et al* (1993)	Hong Kong	7229	DIS	2.78% (m) 0.53% (f)
Levav *et al* (1993)	Israel	2741	SADS–I	0.7%
Kessler *et al* (1994)	US (NCS)	8098	CIDI	3.5%
Samuels *et al* (1994)	US	810	DSM–III rating scale	1.5%

SADS, Schedule for Affective Disorders and Schizophrenia (SADS–L, Lifetime version; SADS–I, Israel version); SIB, Schedule for Interviewing Borderlines; DIS, Diagnostic Interview Schedule; PDQ, Personality Disorders Questionnaire; SIDP, Structured Interview for DSM–III Personality Disorders; SCID, Structured Clinical Interview for DSM–III–R Personality Disorders; CIDI, Composite International Diagnostic Interview; ECA, Epidemiological Catchment Area; NCS, National Comorbidity Survey.

Methodological considerations

The findings from the reviewed studies included in Tables 2.1 and 2.2 should be considered in the light of the methodology employed. Some of the more important methodological issues will be considered under the following headings: case definition, sampling decisions, and reporting of the results.

Case definition

A major problem facing epidemiological investigators has been that of diagnosis. All of the studies included in Table 2.1 relied upon clinical judgement (in some shape or form) in order to define caseness. For example, the Essen-Moller (1956) study relied upon a psychiatrist personally interviewing every member of the study population or a sample thereof. The Leighton (1959) study involved the application of clinical judgements to data collected by assistants. It is now generally agreed that this approach is unsatisfactory. Clinical judgements are rarely sufficiently explicit to be stated in operational terms and often lack consistency in the criteria applied for making a diagnosis (Kreitman, 1993). Independent replication therefore becomes almost impossible.

The development of standardised diagnostic criteria and the accompanying standard interviews has partially remedied the problems of consistency in case definition. The majority of studies listed in Table 2.2 have relied on the Diagnostic Interview Schedule (DIS; Robins *et al*, 1981,) as case detector. The DIS is a highly structured interview designed for use by specially trained interviewers. It collects data sufficient for making a diagnosis by three systems: DSM–III, the Feighner criteria (Feighner *et al*, 1972) and the Research Diagnostic Criteria (RDC; Endicott & Spitzer, 1979). It assesses symptoms which may have occurred at any time during the patient's life, and in more detail over the previous two weeks, one month, six months and one year. It is possible to use it in the assessment of a variety of mental disorders, although, of the categories of personality disorder, it is only able to detect antisocial personality disorder. A major limitation with the instrument is that it generates findings that rely entirely on retrospective self-report.

There are major inconsistencies in the literature on the psychometric properties of the DIS. Robins *et al* (1981) reported good agreement between a lay interviewer and a psychiatrist for DSM–III diagnoses (mean kappa = 0.69, sensitivity = 0.75, specificity = 0.94). Folstein *et al* (1985), however, found poor agreement between DIS diagnosis and diagnosis obtained by a full psychiatric examination,

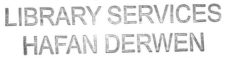

termed clinical reappraisal: sensitivity (i.e. the proportion of clinical reappraisal cases also identified by DIS) for antisocial personality disorder = 0.26; specificity (i.e. the proportion of clinical reappraisal non-cases also found to be non-cases by DIS) = 0.99. These results suggest that the DIS may grossly underestimate the number of cases of antisocial personality disorder. In contrast, Perry *et al* (1987) found that DIS and clinical diagnoses of antisocial personality disorder agreed well (sensitivity = 0.95. specificity = 0.7). Such serious inconsistencies raise doubts about the validity of the DIS.

Kessler *et al* (1994) used the Composite International Diagnostic Interview (CIDI) as case detector. This is a structured diagnostic interview based on the DIS and designed to be used by trained lay interviewers. Field trials of the CIDI have thus far documented good reliability and validity (Wittchen *et al*, 1991), although there is less experience with the CIDI compared with the DIS and it remains to be seen whether these good psychometric properties will be replicated in further studies.

Weissman & Myers (1980) relied on the Schedule for Affective Disorders and Schizophrenia (Lifetime Version) (SADS–L) as case detector. Levav *et al* (1993) used a modified Israeli version of the same instrument (SADS–I) in order to generate six-month and lifetime prevalence rates of mental disorder. The SADS–L is a structured interview which was designed for use with hospital patients, and not designed for use in a community survey. Nevertheless, it is a highly reliable instrument when used by specially trained workers. It is only able to detect and diagnose antisocial and borderline disorders, which it does according to Research Diagnostic Criteria (RDC). A higher threshold is required to diagnose RDC antisocial personality than is required for DSM–III. This may explain the consistently lower rates of antisocial personality disorder obtained by the SADS–L in community studies of antisocial personality disorder.

Zimmerman & Coryell (1990) examined not only the prevalence of personality disorders in a community sample, but were also able to test the comparability of two instruments. They interviewed 697 relatives of psychiatric patients and healthy controls with the Structured Interview for DSM–III Personality Disorders (SIDP) and the Personality Disorders Questionnaire (PDQ). The SIDP is a highly structured interview with the patient or an informant, and the PDQ is a much briefer self-report questionnaire. The authors found poor agreement between the instruments when the scores were analysed categorically, although the dimensional scores were far better correlated. They concluded that the SIDP provided the best estimate of the prevalence of antisocial personality disorder, and that the PDQ was more vulnerable to a response set bias and failed to assess some items comprehensively.

Sampling decisions

Antisocial personality disorder is not very common and therefore, in order to ensure that sufficient numbers are detected, epidemiological studies require either very large samples or high-risk populations. All the studies listed in Table 2.2 follow this principle. For example, the Epidemiological Catchment Area (ECA) programme (Robins & Regier, 1991) sampled at least 3500 subjects from five geographical sites, giving a total sample size of over 18 000. Zimmerman & Coryell (1990) and Baron *et al* (1985) recruited first-degree relatives of psychiatric patients – genetic research indicates that this group is likely to be at high risk for personality disorders (McGuffin & Thapar, 1993).

Non-response is a fundamental problem for all epidemiological research because it can lead to significant bias in the estimation of rates of a disorder. On account of the fact that antisocial subjects are by definition non-cooperative and non-compliant, it is likely that refusal rates will be particularly high among this group. The magnitude of this problem is compounded by the fact that, in general, there has been a secular decrease in survey response rates since the 1950s (Lloyd & Weich, 1997).

The chaotic lifestyle associated with antisocial personality disorder, characterised by frequent changes in job, disrupted relationships and frequent trouble with the law, means that very often epidemiological surveys will have missed a significant number of antisocial subjects – subjects who for the above reasons may go to considerable lengths to avoid any sort of detection. In addition, there is evidence to suggest that individuals with antisocial personality disorder are likely to be particularly mobile, with increased prevalence rates in emigrant groups (Helgason, 1981). These problems lead to high rates of attrition in longitudinal studies, but will inevitably also lead to an underestimation of the baseline prevalence rate in any community survey of antisocial personality disorder.

The denominator in a prevalence calculation requires geographical boundaries, inclusion criteria for age, and definition by type of residence. All of the listed studies in Table 2.2, with the exception of Levav *et al* (1993), sampled household residents over the age of 18 years (the Israeli study included everyone in a birth cohort, regardless of place of residence). Sampling only household residents means that important data on the prevalence of mental disorder in the homeless population will be missed. This information has been obtained in surveys looking directly at the homeless population (e.g. Koegel *et al*, 1988).

No matter how carefully an epidemiological survey is planned, there will always be a discrepancy between the characteristics of the sample obtained and those of the base population. This is the result of sampling error, failure of the sampling frame (e.g. electoral roll) to reflect the real population accurately and non-response. Nevertheless, various sampling strategies can be employed to minimise these sources of error. The majority of the studies listed in Table 2.2 initially drew a sample of addresses, weighted according to household size, and sampled residents from within each address using a grid technique, known as the Kish method (Kish, 1965). Some of the studies have also deliberately oversampled certain subgroups of the population in order to obtain a larger number of cases. Thus, in the ECA study, in order to obtain information pertaining to a possible effect of ethnic status, the non-White population of St Louis (which was in the minority) was oversampled. For similar reasons, the Israeli study oversampled educated members of disadvantaged ethnic groups.

Reporting of results

The results of the studies listed in Table 2.2 are all given as lifetime prevalence rates. Lifetime prevalence of a disorder is defined as the proportion of persons in a representative sample of the population who have ever experienced that disorder up to the date of assessment. It is one of the few measures that can be estimated solely on the basis of a single personal interview in a cross-sectional survey. It can provide useful information about the aetiology of a disorder because it identifies a larger number of cases than does point or period prevalence. However, there are also certain drawbacks in using lifetime prevalence in the assessment of the frequency of a disorder. First, if a disorder carries with it an increased risk of death, rates in older persons will have been reduced by mortality more than rates in younger persons, as they have survived a longer period of risk for increased mortality than younger persons. This can create the false impression that the rate of the disorder is increasing in younger generations. This may be particularly relevant when considering the age distribution of antisocial personality disorder.

Second, there is the problem of impaired recall. The assessment of lifetime prevalence using an instrument such as the DIS or SADS–L relies on the ability to assess psychiatric status historically. Although no psychiatric interview will be impervious to errors in recall, compared with a lay interviewer who administers the DIS, a psychiatrist has more training in picking up clues that a denied symptom may exist, and has a greater variety of techniques with which to prompt recall. It is not clear how much these techniques improve the accuracy of self-report.

The main findings of the studies listed in Table 2.2 will now be discussed, in the light of the above considerations.

Main findings from community surveys

Antisocial personality disorder is recognised and found in all societies (Murphy, 1976), although there are important cross-cultural differences in prevalence. It should be noted that antisocial personality disorder has been the only axis II disorder to have been systematically studied in all community surveys of psychiatric morbidity. Before comparing the lifetime prevalence rates listed in Table 2.2, it should be emphasised that the studies employed a variety of methods of data collection and a variety of diagnostic criteria (e.g. RDC, DSM) were used. The rates vary from 0.14% in Taiwan to 3.7% in Canada, with the majority of studies falling between 2 and 3% of the population sampled. The low rate in Taiwan is in keeping with the lower rates of most DSM–III disorders as measured by the DIS in the Taiwan site. (The only disorders that have considerably higher rates in Taiwan, as compared with the rest of the world reporting data, are generalised anxiety and tobacco use disorders.) A possible explanation for the considerably lower rate of antisocial personality disorder in Taiwan is that there may be a higher threshold for the reporting of antisocial behaviour in Taiwan (i.e. a response bias). Compton *et al* (1991) have looked specifically at cross-cultural differences in the rates of antisocial personality disorder by comparing ECA data with those from the Taiwan Psychiatric Epidemiological Project. They concluded that while the considerably lower rate of disorder in Taiwan might be partially attributable to response bias, this was unlikely to explain the whole magnitude of difference. The low prevalence in Taiwan does not, however, translate to other East Asian countries; rates in Hong Kong and South Korea are comparable with those in Europe and the US. These countries also have very high rates of alcoholism, and literature from psychiatric settings indicates a clear association between the two conditions (Ross, 1995; Tomasson & Vaglum, 1995).

Consistently lower rates are obtained in surveys using the PDQ and the SADS–L. The lower rates obtained using the PDQ (Reich *et al*, 1989; Zimmerman & Coryell, 1990) highlight the fact that use of self-report may lead to an underestimation of the prevalence of antisocial personality disorder. As mentioned previously, the higher threshold of symptoms required for making a diagnosis of antisocial personality disorder using the SADS–L may explain the low rates obtained in Israel and two of the American sites. (The finding from Israel is particularly surprising in the light of the cohort design employed, which allowed the investigators to trace some cohort members into prisons. The addition of a forensic population to what was ostensibly a community sample should have raised the community prevalence rate to an artificially high level. The fact that this did not occur suggests that the SADS–I may have been under-reporting.)

Demographic correlates

If the results of the studies are examined in greater detail, some clear demographic correlates of antisocial personality disorder emerge.

Gender

In all of the studies listed, males are affected much more frequently than females. In the ECA study, the average gender ratio of men to women was 6:1. Swanson *et al* (1994), reporting on data obtained from Bland *et al*'s (1988) study, found a ratio of 8:1. Although there was a trend in the New Zealand data (Wells *et al*, 1989), it failed to reach statistical significance, which the authors attributed to inadequate sample size leading to lack of power. Similarly, there were no significant gender differences reported in Taiwan (Hwu *et al*, 1989), although the trend was in the same direction. There is very little literature on the characteristics of women with antisocial personality disorder. Mulder *et al* (1994) compared the demographic and clinical characteristics of 22 women with antisocial personality disorder with a community sample of women without the disorder and 22 men with antisocial personality disorder. Compared with the other two samples, women with antisocial personality disorder had higher rates of marital separation, chronic unemployment and dependence on the state. They also had high rates of comorbid psychiatric disorder and frequently used psychiatric services.

Age

In all of the studies, antisocial personality disorder prevalence rates declined with age. In the ECA study, rates were consistently higher in the age group 25–44 years. Between 45 and 64 years rates declined dramatically. Similar findings were reported in New Zealand, Canada, Germany, Hong Kong, Korea and Taiwan. Swanson *et al* (1994) reported an almost perfect correlation between age and remission rate (0.98). Some authors (Robins, 1985; Paris, 1997*a*) have cited this as evidence for a rising rate of antisocial personality disorder. Robins (1985) supports this argument with the finding that violent crime is increasing (Welford, 1973). Until a clearer understanding of the natural history of the disorder exists, and in the light of the pitfalls associated with lifetime prevalence rates, the age-related epidemiological findings are best interpreted with caution.

Urban/rural differences

The effect of urbanisation is less clear than the age and gender effects. Not all of the listed studies looked for an effect, and in those that did there are inconsistencies in the size of the effect reported. The ECA study (Robins & Regier, 1991) found that for the St Louis site the rate of antisocial personality disorder was approximately twice as high for the inner-city sample as for residents of a small town and rural area (5.7 v. 2.4%). The Korean study (Lee *et al*, 1990) found a significantly greater prevalence of antisocial personality disorder in urban Seoul compared with rural areas (2.08 v. 0.91%). In contrast, the National Comorbidity Survey (Kessler *et al*, 1994) did not confirm an urban/rural difference, although it found that antisocial personality disorder was more common in the Western states of the USA, a difference which it has been suggested may be due to the migration of antisocial individuals (Paris, 1997*a*).

Socio-economic status

The National Comorbidity Survey has been the only study of those listed to have adequately assessed socio-economic status. A dramatic decline in the rate of antisocial personality disorder was found as income increased (odds ratio for income bracket US$0–19 000: 2.98; odds ratio for income bracket >US$70 000: 1.00).

Marital status

Of the listed studies, only Bland *et al* (1988*a*) specifically examined lifetime prevalence of antisocial personality disorder by marital status. The highest rate was found in the widowed, separated and divorced, and the lowest rate was found in the married.

Education

Three studies specifically examined the effect of educational status on prevalence rate. The ECA study found that rates of antisocial personality disorder were lower in college graduates than in non-graduates. The National Comorbidity Survey looked at the effect in greater detail and found that for those leaving formal education at age 11 years, the odds ratio for antisocial personality disorder was 14.1 (95% CI 6.1–33.0); for those remaining in education until 15 years, the odds ratio was 3.3 (95% CI 1.4–7.7). Finally, Levav *et al* (1993) noted that the six-month prevalence rate for antisocial personality disorder declined from 0.66% in those subjects with less than high school education to 0.25% in those who had received high school education.

Race

Neither the ECA study (which examined 'Black' and 'non-Black' subjects) nor the National Comorbidity Survey (which examined 'Black', 'White' and 'Hispanic' subjects) detected any significant differences in the rates of antisocial personality disorder with respect to race. The Israeli study found that rates of antisocial personality disorder were significantly higher in Israelis of North African origin than in those of European origin. These results may reflect the lower social status of North African Israelis.

Frequency of symptoms

Swanson *et al* (1994) and Robins (1985) examined the frequency of symptoms of DSM–III antisocial personality disorder in community samples. Swanson's group found that the most common symptoms were job troubles (91.3%), physical violence (83.7%), traffic offences (81.7%), childhood thefts (76%), school truancy (73.1%), childhood violations at home/school (70.2%) and relationship problems (60.6%). All other symptoms occurred in less than 60% of antisocial personality disorder subjects. The ECA study found an overall lower frequency of symptoms. The most common symptoms were: fighting (78%), job troubles (70%), promiscuity (61%) and traffic offences (56%); all other symptoms occurred at a frequency of less than 50% of subjects.

Studies in primary care

Psychological problems in the primary health care setting constitute a major public health problem (Sartorius *et al*, 1993). Although there is a large literature on the form and frequency of mental disorders in primary care, comparatively few studies have examined the epidemiology of personality disorders in this setting. In particular, little is known about the prevalence of antisocial personality disorder. In addition, the categories of personality disorder recognised by the current classification systems have been developed largely from studies of psychiatric patients, and little is known about their utility in primary care.

Studies of unspecified personality disorders

Historically, there has been a tradition for classifying personality disorders under the broad heading of neurosis, making it impossible to estimate specific rates of personality disorders. The majority of contemporary studies that have distinguished personality disorder from neurosis have only looked at rates of unspecified personality disorders.

All identified studies that have looked at the prevalence of unspecified personality disorders in primary care are listed in Table 2.3. The tabulated studies indicate that in representative samples of primary care attenders, 5–8% are identified as having an unspecified personality disorder. This figure rises to over 30% in samples selected with psychiatric disturbance. This dramatic rise may reflect a genuine increase in the rate of personality disorder, or alternatively may be an artefact due to state effects. Four of the 12 studies included did not use a standardised instrument in the assessment of personality, and for this reason the reliability of the prevalence rates obtained is questionable. The importance of using a structured interview in the assessment of abnormal personality has been demonstrated by Casey *et al* (1984). In this study, the personality of every patient with conspicuous psychiatric morbidity was examined by clinical interview and with the Personality Assessment Schedule (PAS; Tyrer *et al*, 1979). A personality disorder was diagnosed by the general practitioner as the primary diagnosis in 8.9% and by a research psychiatrist in 6.4% of subjects. These figures rose to 33.9% when a subject was formally assessed with the PAS. Six of the 12 studies used selected samples of patients, and it is unclear how safely the findings can be generalised to routine general practice.

Studies of antisocial personality disorder

Although the literature search revealed only three studies that looked specifically at the prevalence of antisocial personality disorder in primary care (Schulberg *et al*, 1985; Smith *et al*, 1991; Sato & Takeichi, 1993), two of the tabulated studies produced findings relevant to the epidemiology of antisocial personality disorder. Casey *et al* (1984) found that among a sample of primary care attenders with conspicuous psychiatric morbidity, the most common personality disorder was explosive. Similarly, in a more representative sample of 200 primary care attenders in which the frequency of personality disorder was 13%, explosive personality disorder was the most common (Casey & Tyrer, 1986). Although this now-deleted ICD–9 category specifically excluded dissocial personality, the aggression criterion that featured in the ICD–9 glossary description is entirely congruent with the current ICD–10 concept of dissocial personality disorder.

TABLE 2.3
Surveys of unspecified personality disorder carried out in primary care

Author	Location	Sample	Procedure	Findings
Kessel (1960)	1 suburban UK general practice	911 randomly selected patients	Clinical interview	5% prevalence rate 'abnormal personality'
Cooper (1965)	10 UK general practices	100 patients with 'chronic psychiatric disorder'	Clinical interview	8% identified by psychiatrist as having personality disorder
Cooper (1972)	8 UK general practices	115 selected patients with psychiatric disorder	Clinical interview using ICD–8 criteria	6% prevalence rate personality disorder m=7.1% f=5.7%
Mann *et al* (1981)	2 UK general practices	87 patients with non-psychotic disorder identified by GP	SAP with 12-month follow-up	31/87 had abnormal personalities. At 12-month follow-up consumption of psychotropics associated with personality abnormality
Casey *et al* (1984)	UK inner-city general practice	171 patients referred by GP suffering from psychiatric disturbance	PAS	33.9% point prevalence unspecified personality disorder; explosive most frequent
Kessler (1985)	Primary care clinic in Wisconsin, US	192 randomly selected patients	SADS–L One-year follow-up study	Of 'continuing cases' of psychiatric disorder 33.3% had labile personality disorder

contd...

TABLE 2.3 (*contd...*)

Casey & Tyrer (1986)	2 UK general practices: 1 urban, 1 rural	200 randomly selected patients	PAS	13% point prevalence unspecified personality disorder; explosive most frequent; urban=rural
Barrett *et al* (1988)	Rural general practice in US	260 consecutive attenders	SADS	1.3% had a 'labile personality'
Dilling *et al* (1989)	18 general practices in Upper Bavaria	1274 randomly selected patients	CIS and ICD–8 criteria	9.4% prevalence rate personality disorder
Casey & Tyrer (1990)	2 UK general practices: 1 urban, 1 rural	358 patients with psychiatric morbidity	PAS	28% 1-year prevalence unspecified personality disorder; urban > rural
Ceroni *et al* (1992)	11 general practices in Northern Italy	66 consecutive attenders	Clinical interview	12.1% point prevalence 'personality disorder'
Patience *et al* (1995)	14 Scottish general practices	113 patients with DSM–III major depression	PAS treatment study: random allocation to 1 of 4 treatments with PAS administered after improvement	26% prevalence rate personality disorder Presence of personality pathology delayed recovery from depression

SAP, Standardised Assessment of Personality; PAS, Personality Assessment Schedule; SADS, Schedule for Affective Disorders and Schizophrenia (SADS–L, Lifetime version); CIS, Clinical Interview Schedule.

In a study whose primary intention was to assess the efficiency of detecting depression in primary care, Schulberg *et al* (1985) interviewed 294 primary medical care patients with the DIS and established a prevalence rate for antisocial personality disorder of 5.8%. The authors did not comment on this finding, which is surprisingly high given that approximately 70% of the interview subjects were women. The findings might be explained by the fact that a disproportionate number of young subjects were sampled, and as such this study was not looking at a representative group of primary care attenders.

In order to test an association between antisocial personality disorder and somatisation disorder, Smith *et al* (1991) interviewed 118 primary care patients suffering from somatisation disorder, using the DIS and the SCID–II. Prevalence rates for antisocial personality disorder were 8.2% for women and 25% for men. The authors concluded that the data were consistent with a hypothesised association between the two disorders. Using a two-stage method of case identification (General Health Questionnaire followed by DIS), Sato & Takeichi (1993) were unable to identify any cases of antisocial personality disorder among a sample of 172 randomly selected Japanese primary care attenders. The authors attributed this finding to culture-specific factors, such as a higher threshold for reporting antisocial symptoms and possibly the existence of fewer socio-demographic risk factors for the development of antisocial personality disorder in Japanese society. Honda (1983) has also pointed out that the types of personality disorders described in DSM–III are unfamiliar to Japanese psychiatrists.

Studies carried out in psychiatric settings

In their review of studies of personality disorder carried out in psychiatric settings, de Girolamo & Reich (1993) concluded:

> "While it is clear that the prevalence of personality disorders among psychiatric outpatients and inpatients may be high ... it is not possible to reach any conclusion on the basis of the available studies, as the prevalence rates found are very different. These differences are related to differences in sampling, diagnostic methods employed, coverage and accessibility of mental health services and a variety of other sociocultural factors."

Little has changed in the literature since 1993. Epidemiological studies of personality disorder subtypes within selected samples of psychiatric patients continue to proliferate (particularly those of borderline personality disorder). As will be evident later, prevalence studies of antisocial personality disorder in certain selected samples, for example drug users, may give rise to inflated estimates of the prevalence of the disorder in psychiatric settings. A more balanced picture of distribution in this setting is gleaned from studies of unselected admissions to hospital, and Table 2.4 lists some of the main studies of the prevalence of antisocial personality disorder in samples of unselected psychiatric patients. (Studies of patients from specialist treatment settings, such as the Henderson Hospital (e.g. Dolan & Mitchell, 1994) not unexpectedly report high prevalence rates for personality disorders and do not yield a representative picture; for this reason they have been omitted from this section.)

It is clear, from first inspection, that the number of prevalence studies in unselected samples of psychiatric patients is comparatively few compared with the burgeoning number of so-called comorbidity studies. There are too few studies using too many different methods to draw any firm conclusions about the prevalence of antisocial personality disorder/dissocial personality disorder in general psychiatric settings. It does, however, seem that antisocial personality disorder/dissocial personality disorder is a comparatively rare category of personality disorder in general psychiatric settings. Epidemiological studies indicate that in general psychiatric settings the most common type of personality disorder is borderline personality disorder (De Girolamo & Reich, 1993).

The majority of the listed studies quote prevalence rates of between 1 and 3% for antisocial personality disorder. Notable exceptions are Alnaes & Torgesen's (1988) finding of no cases of antisocial personality disorder in their sample of consecutive out-patients, and Dahl's rate of 18.2%. Alnaes & Torgesen excluded patients with "mainly social problems" and substance misuse – two groups which could be expected to contain large numbers of cases of antisocial personality disorder. Dahl's finding is in keeping with the prevalence rates quoted for other cluster B disorders and is something of an anomaly by comparison with the remaining studies.

The studies of Cutting *et al* (1986) and Jackson *et al* (1991) both selected patients with serious mental illness and are not strictly studies of unselected samples, although in defence of their inclusion is the fact that they did not limit their selection to a single diagnostic category as so many other studies have done. Cutting *et al* examined the prevalence of abnormal personality traits in a group of patients with schizophrenia, affective disorder and other functional psychoses. Jackson *et al* examined prevalence rates of personality disorders in a similar mixed group of patients. Both studies found an association with schizophrenia.

TABLE 2.4
Surveys of the prevalence of antisocial personality disorder (and diagnostic equivalents) in psychiatric patients

Author	Country	Sample	Method of assessment	Findings
Kass *et al* (1985)	US	609 new consecutive out-patients	DSM–III rating scale	51% of patients had a personality disorder Prevalence of antisocial personality disorder=2%
Koenigsberg *et al* (1985)	US	2462 patients from out-patient clinic, in-patient unit, 'walk-in' clinic and consultation–liaison service	Clinical diagnosis	36% of patients had a personality disorder Prevalence of antisocial personality disorder=2%
Cutting *et al* (1986)	UK	100 consecutive admissions with major affective disorder or psychosis	SAP	44% of patients had abnormal personality 3% had sociopathic traits
Dahl (1986)	Norway	103 consecutive admissions to hospital	SADS	45% of patients had a personality disorder Prevalence of antisocial personality disorder=18.2%
Alnaes & Torgesen (1988)	Norway	298 consecutive out-patients	SIDP	81% of patients had a personality disorder No cases of antisocial personality disorder found
Pilgrim & Mann (1990)	UK	120 consecutive new admissions to psychiatric hospital	SAP	36% of patients had a personality disorder Prevalence of dissocial personality disorder=1.6%
Jackson *et al* (1991)	Australia	112 in-patients	SIDP	46% of patients had a personality disorder Antisocial personality disorder occurred in 20% of people with schizophrenia and 15% of people with mania
Oldham *et al* (1995)	US	200 consecutive applicants for in-patient care or psychotherapy	SCID–II PDE	3.5% antisocial personality disorder

SAP, Standardised Assessment of Personality; SADS, Schedule for Affective Disorders and Schizophrenia (SADS–L, Lifetime version); SIDP, Structured Interview for DSM–III Personality Disorders; SCID–II, Structured Clinical Interview for DSM–III–R Personality Disorders; PDE, Personality Disorder Examination.

Hospital admission data

Another relevant source of information on the epidemiology of antisocial personality disorder in psychiatric settings is hospital admission data. Brooke (1980) has criticised the use of health service statistics as a source of epidemiological data on the grounds that they are incomplete, overemphasise in-patient activity and are heavily dependent on a clinician's personal diagnosis, as recorded in a summary sheet. Nevertheless, despite such limitations, national statistics have the considerable advantage of availability (Mann, 1993).

Using hospital admission data, Mulder (1991) carried out a survey of all in-patients admitted to psychiatric hospitals in New Zealand over a seven-year period with a primary ICD–9 diagnosis of a personality disorder. Over the seven-year period there were 6447 admissions with a primary diagnosis of personality disorder. The most common category was unspecified personality disorder (45%). This was followed by dependent (12%), sociopathic (10%), histrionic (9%), explosive (6%), schizoid (5%), other (5%), paranoid (3%), affective (3%), and anankastic personality disorders (2%). The majority of sociopathic patients were young (<24 years) unmarried men, involuntarily admitted to hospital.

The Department of Health Hospital Episode Statistics system records numbers of finished consultant episodes with a mental illness diagnosis. The numbers of finished consultant episodes for sociopathic personality disorder between 1989 and 1995 are given in Table 2.5.

A finished consultant episode is an episode where the patient has completed a period of care under one consultant within one hospital provider and is transferred to another consultant, is discharged, or has died. (An admission is where the patient has entered a hospital

TABLE 2.5
Proportion of 'finished consultant episodes' (FCEs) with any mention of sociopathic personality disorder (ICD–9 301.7), 1989–1995. (Source: Hospital Episode Statistics (Department of Health) by personal communication, 1998)

Year	FCEs with any mention of sociopathic personality disorder (n)	FCEs with a primary diagnosis of mental illness (ICD–9 290–319) (n)	%
1989–90	1000	301 810	0.33
1990–91	1140	304 960	0.37
1991–92	1130	305 840	0.37
1992–93	1370	313 210	0.44
1993–94	1270	313 900	0.40
1994–95	1200	317 290	0.38

and is placed under the care of a consultant. A count of admissions during a year would include finished and unfinished episodes, i.e. those patients who had been admitted during the year and were still in hospital.) As can be seen, sociopathic personality disorder constitutes a small but relatively constant proportion of total finished consultant episodes (about 0.3–0.5%).

There is evidence from studies of hospital admission rates that diagnostic changes have a significant effect on the overall prevalence rate of patients with personality disorders in contact with psychiatric services. Simonsen & Mellergard (1988) analysed data concerning admissions to psychiatric institutions in Denmark in the years 1975, 1980 and 1985. A diagnosis of borderline personality disorder increased in prevalence from 5 to 20%. This paralleled a decrease in the prevalence of a diagnosis of psychopathy from 22 to 7%. Although the changes may be coincidental, the authors suggested that one explanation might be that those patients previously diagnosed as psychopaths are now being diagnosed as having borderline personality disorder.

Studies carried out in prison settings

The accurate determination of the prevalence rate of mental disorder in prison settings is considerably difficult. Several factors significantly affect the estimation of prevalence, making comparison of estimates between prison systems extremely difficult. These factors include the location of the study (European and American courts operate quite differently), the type of prison (sentenced or remand), the type of prisoner studied (according to gender, type of offence, type of sentence or stage of sentence) and a variety of other factors that determine the actual numbers of mentally disordered offenders entering the criminal justice system at any point in time. These include: the prevalence of mental disorder in the community; police practices in diverting suspects judged to be mentally disordered to hospitals; and the operation of court diversion schemes. When one considers these factors in the light of the difficulties involved in the assessment of personality disorders, it is clear that estimation of the prevalence of antisocial personality disorder in prison settings is going to be fraught with potential problems.

Coid (1984) has comprehensively reviewed the literature on the prevalence of psychiatric morbidity in prison populations over this century. Studies that attempted to obtain a random or otherwise representative sample of the overall prison population were included. Retrospective studies, and those using non-random sampling procedures, were excluded. Only 11 studies met Coid's criteria for inclusion, five from the US and five from the UK. Eight of the studies from Coid's review estimated the prevalence of psychopathy/personality disorder, and these are presented in Table 2.6. Most of the studies based their sample on single prisons (usually local prisons) which are not representative of the entire prison estate. Sampling decisions varied considerably, with some studies conducting a virtual census of the entire population over a period of time (Jones, 1976) and others attempting to obtain a random sample of prisoners (Gunn *et al*, 1978). Only three of the tabulated studies made use of standardised diagnoses: Feighner's criteria in Guze (1976), ICD–9 in Gunn *et al* (1978) and DSM–II in Jones (1976). There are inconsistencies in the terminology used, and this complicates the

TABLE 2.6
Sentenced population studies up until 1983 (adapted from Coid, 1984)

Author	Location	Sample	Procedure	Findings
Gluek (1918)	Sing Sing Prison, USA	600 consecutive male receptions	Clinical interview	Psychopathy 18.0%
Roper (1950, 1951)	Wakefield Prison, UK	1100 males, consecutive mixed sentences	Clinical interview, Raven's Progressive Matrices	Psychopathy 8%
Bluglass (1966)	Perth Prison, Scotland	300 males, every 4th reception	Clinical interview	Personality disorder 13%
Faulk (1976)	Winchester Prison, UK	72 males, consecutive releases, mixed sentence	Clinical interview	Alcoholic and personality disorder 75%
Jones (1976)	Tennessee State Penitentiary, Nashville, US	1040 males, entire population	Screened for illness; case notes; DSM–II diagnosis	Personality disorder 5.5%
Guze (1976)	Missouri Probation Board, US	223 male parolees and flat-timers; 66 females	Clinical interview, Feighner's criteria	Sociopathy: males = 78% females = 68%
Gunn *et al* (1978)	South East Prisons Survey, UK	106 males, random sample, 3 security grades	Clinical interview using ICD–9 diagnoses	Personality disorder 22%
James *et al* (1980)	Oklahoma Prison, US	174 males, stratified sample	Clinical interview, self-report score	Personality disorder 35%

process of comparing prevalence rates. Four of the studies quote prevalence rates for 'personality disorder', two of the studies quote 'psychopathy', one study quotes 'alcoholic and personality disorder' and one study quotes 'sociopathy'. For these reasons, it would be unwise to draw any firm conclusions about the distribution of antisocial personality disorder or psychopathy in prisons based on the studies in Table 2.6.

Sentenced population studies: 1983–1996

The main sentenced population studies that included an assessment of personality disorder/antisocial personality disorder/psychopathy and which were published after 1983 are listed in Table 2.7. A significant number of published studies were not included in this table. Reasons for exclusion included lack of a randomised sample (Taylor, 1986; Chiles *et al*, 1990), use of a consecutive reception sample (which introduces bias towards prisoners serving short sentences) (Daniel *et al*, 1988), use of a selected non-representative sample of prisoners (Glaser, 1985), use of mixed remand/sentenced populations (Hurley & Dunne, 1991; Mitchison *et al*, 1994) and inadequate methods of case detection (Glaser, 1985; Taylor, 1986).

It can be seen from Table 2.7 that there have been considerable improvements in methodology. All of the listed studies used standardised assessment procedures, and in contrast to Coid's findings, all of the studies, with the exception of Jordan *et al* (1996), used random samples of prisoners. (Jordan's study was a virtual census of women felons who entered prison over a 17-month period.) There remains, however, a lack of uniformity in the terminology used: all studies from North America quote prevalence rates for antisocial personality disorder or psychopathy, whereas the studies from the UK confine their estimates to 'personality disorder'. The literature search was unable to identify any published estimates of psychopathy/antisocial personality disorder in English prison samples (with the exception of a subsample of disruptive male prisoners in Coid (1992) where the prevalence of SCID-defined antisocial personality disorder was 86% and high-score PCL-defined psychopathy was 77%). Theoretically, the construct of antisocial personality disorder should encompass a narrower group of subjects compared with 'personality disorder', and as such the English studies only provide a coarse proxy measure of the prevalence of antisocial personality disorder. Cooke's Scottish study has adopted the American approach and has quoted rates for trichotomised bands of psychopathy.

TABLE 2.7
Sentenced population studies since 1983

Author	Location	Sample	Procedure	Findings
Hare (1983)	2 Canadian prison populations: (a) federal medium-secure unit; (b) provincial prison	246 White male inmates	PCL, clinical interview using DSM–III criteria	Point prevalence rate of antisocial personality disorder for sample: (a) 33.3%; (b) 41.5% Overall prevalence of antisocial personality disorder 39%
Côté & Hodgins (1990)	Sample of Quebec penitentiaries	Random sample of 650 male inmates	DIS	Lifetime prevalence rate of DSM–III antisocial personality disorder 61.5%
Bland *et al* (1990)	2 correctional centres in Edmonton, Canada	Random sample of 180 male inmates and 1006 age-matched controls	DIS	Lifetime prevalence rate of DSM–III antisocial personality disorder 57% (standardised prevalence ratio x7 general population)
Gunn *et al* (1991)	UK: 16 prisons for adult males; 9 institutions for young male offenders	Random 5% sample of sentenced male population	Clinical interview using ICD–9 criteria Items of CIS Case records	Prevalence rate of personality disorder 10% (*n*=1884)
Côté & Hodgins (1992)	Sample of Quebec penitentiaries	87 homicide convictions selected from 1990 study	DIS	No significant difference in frequency of antisocial personality disorder

contd...

TABLE 2.7 (*contd...*)

Author	Location	Sample	Procedure	Findings
Cooke (1994)	8 Scottish prisons	Stratified sample of 60 female prisoners and 247 male prisoners	SADS–L PCL–R	Males: 15% moderate levels and 3% high levels Females: 7% moderate or high levels of psychopathy
Maden *et al* (1994)	4 prisons in UK	Random sample of 301 women prisoners (25% of sentenced female population)	Semi-structured interview using ICD–9 criteria Items of CIS Case notes	Prevalence rate of personality disorder 18%
Swinton *et al* (1994)	See Gunn *et al* (1991)	170 male life-sentenced prisoners and 1630 non-lifers	See Gunn *et al* (1991)	Prevalence rate of personality disorder: lifers, 18.2%; non-lifers, 7.4%
Jordan *et al* (1996)	Correctional institution for women, Raleigh, NC	Unselected 'census' of all women entering prison over 14 months (*n*=805)	DIS CIDI DIPD	Lifetime prevalence rate of DSM–III–R antisocial personality disorder 11.9%

PCL, Psychopathy Checklist (PCL–R, Revised version); DIS, Diagnostic Interview Schedule; CIS, Clinical Interview Schedule; SADS–L, Schedule for Affective Disorders and Schizophrenia – Lifetime version; CIDI, Composite International Diagnostic Interview; DIPD, Diagnostic Interview for Personality Disorder.

Despite the methodological improvements, only two of the 10 listed studies (Côté & Hodgins, 1990; Bland *et al*, 1990) provide comparable data on the prevalence of antisocial personality disorder in prison settings. Both used random samples of male inmates, the DIS as a case detector, and quote lifetime prevalence rates for antisocial personality disorder of the order of 60%. (Hodgins (1995) criticised the use of the DIS in prison populations and suggested that the prevalence figures obtained with it underestimate the true prevalence of mental disorder.) Interestingly, the UK data have produced much more conservative estimates for the prevalence of personality disorder (approximately 10%) – a term which encompasses a broader range of psychopathology. Therefore, there appears to be a dramatic cross-cultural difference in the rate of antisocial personality disorder. This difference probably reflects the very low symptom threshold required to diagnose DSM–III antisocial personality disorder, together with the factors influencing admission rates mentioned above.

Hare (1983) sought not only to determine the prevalence of antisocial personality disorder in two prisons, but also to compare the agreement between DSM–III antisocial personality disorder and a PCL-defined rating of psychopathy. Overall, 39% of the prisoners received a diagnosis of antisocial personality disorder. Good agreement was found between a diagnosis of DSM–III antisocial personality disorder and PCL scores (kappa = 0.83).

Côté & Hodgins' study provides interesting data on co-occurring mental disorders in prisoners. They found that of the 303 inmates with antisocial personality disorder, 73% had between one and two additional lifetime diagnoses. The disorder most strongly associated with antisocial personality disorder was drug misuse (odds ratio for having a diagnosis of drug misuse given a diagnosis of antisocial personality disorder = 3.09), a consistent finding in the literature. A subsample of homicide offenders was also looked at (Côté & Hodgins, 1992). No significant increase in the prevalence of antisocial personality disorder was found in the homicide group.

Bland *et al* (1990) is the only study of those listed in Table 2.7 to employ a community control group, and as such is the only one which allows a direct comparison to be made between prison and community prevalence. By calculating the Standardised Prevalence Ratio (ratio of observed to expected numbers of cases), the authors were able to establish directly that the prevalence rate of antisocial personality disorder in the prison setting was almost seven times that found in the general population. (It should be emphasised that the vast majority of prison surveys have found that the rates of almost all mental disorders among inmates in prisons far exceed rates for these disorders in the general population. In the majority of cases, the major disorder is present before the current period of incarceration.)

Gunn *et al* (1991) assessed not only the prevalence of ICD–9 mental disorder in a representative 5% sample of the sentenced male population, but also determined the psychiatric 'treatment needs' of the assessed population and provided a natural link between the literature on epidemiology and needs assessment. Diagnostic status was determined by the use of a semi-structured interview and supplemented with information from case files. A standardised assessment tool was not used to assess personality, and the authors acknowledge that their method is likely to underdiagnose personality disorders. This fact may account for the unexpectedly low rate of personality disorders obtained in the study (10%).

Cooke's (1994) study of Scottish prisons used trichotomised PCL scores to determine what proportion of prisoners were psychopaths. Only 7% of the female sample were regarded as having either moderate or high levels of psychopathy. Of the males, 15% had moderate levels of psychopathy, whereas only 3% were in the high category. Cooke contrasted these findings with those of Hare (1991) in Canada, who found that in combined samples of male prison inmates 45% were in the moderate category and 23% in the high category. Cooke also found high levels of association between psychopathy, alcohol and drug dependence. A clear association was also found between psychopathy and violent offending.

Maden *et al* (1994) compared a 25% cross-sectional sample of the sentenced female population with Gunn *et al*'s (1991) 5% sample of the male sentenced population. In contrast to predictions from community surveys about the prevalence of personality disorder in women, the authors found a proportionally higher prevalence rate of personality disorder in female prisoners (odds ratio 1.9; 95% CI 1.4–2.8). Similarly, higher rates of neurosis, drug dependence and learning disability were found. The authors concluded that the most likely explanation for these findings was the low rate of offending in 'normal'/non-personality disordered women.

Swinton *et al* (1994) examined a sample of 170 male life-sentenced prisoners taken from Gunn *et al*'s (1991) cohort. Using a semi-structured interview to generate ICD–9 diagnoses, they found the prevalence of personality disorder to be significantly greater in the life-sentenced population (18.2%; 95% CI 12.4–24) than in the non-lifer population (7.4%; CI 6.1–8.7) with an odds ratio of 2.8 (95% CI 1.8–4.3).

Jordan *et al* (1996) is the only study to provide information on the demographic correlates of the lifetime prevalence of antisocial personality disorder in sentenced female prisoners. It is also the only prison survey to assess the lifetime prevalence of borderline personality disorder in addition to antisocial personality disorder. Instruments used were the CIDI, the DIPD–R, the Revised Diagnostic Interview for Borderlines (DIB–R; Gunderson *et al*, 1981) and the Impact of Events Scale. The most prevalent disorders were drug misuse, borderline personality disorder and antisocial personality disorder. The total prevalence of antisocial personality disorder in the sample was 11.9%, the highest prevalence occurring in poorly educated White city-dwellers aged 18–24 years. The data were compared with old ECA data in order to show that the prevalence of antisocial personality disorder in White women is 15 times higher in prison than in the community. (The authors acknowledge that this comparison should be cautiously interpreted since the ECA data were collected 10 years prior to the inmate data, and the rate differences across studies may reflect, in part, changes in the rates of disorder over time.) Interestingly, the current (six-month) prevalence of borderline personality disorder was over twice that of antisocial personality disorder (28%), suggesting that an important source of morbidity may have been missed by previous prison surveys.

Remand population studies

The remand prison setting is a critical place to gather psychiatric epidemiological data, as it is the penultimate point in the criminal justice process where mentally disordered offenders can be diverted to the health system. As such, the remand setting has been referred to as the first "unfiltered" phase of imprisonment (Andersen *et al*, 1996). In addition, a significant number of prisoners are remanded in custody specifically for the purpose of generating psychiatric reports. For these reasons, one would expect remand prisons to have high rates of mental disorder. Unfortunately, there is a paucity of research in this area. Furthermore, work from the US is not strictly comparable with European studies, because the population on 'remand' (referred to as the 'jail' population) comprises those pretrial and those sentenced to a term of less than one year. All published remand studies that were identified by the literature search and included a measure of the prevalence of antisocial personality disorder/personality disorder are listed in Table 2.8. An attempt has been made only to include American studies that distinguished pre-trial from sentenced prisoners.

In many ways, the literature is in a similar state to that of the sentenced population literature when reviewed by Coid in 1984. Given the paucity of studies in this group, less stringent criteria have been applied in selection for inclusion in the review. Of the 12 studies listed, only three used random samples of prisoners and standardised procedures for assessing caseness (Maden *et al*, 1996;

TABLE 2.8
Remand population studies

Author	Location	Sample	Procedure	Findings
Bowden (1978)	Brixton remand prison	126 men remanded for medical report	Clinical interview generating ICD diagnoses	12% 'psychopathic disorder' (MHA); 24% personality disorder
Taylor & Gunn (1984)	Brixton remand prison	1241 male remand prisoners	Review of prison records using checklist (generating ICD–9 diagnoses)	13.8% personality disorder
Guy *et al* (1985)	Philadelphia prison system	486 male remand prisoners	Clinical interview Variety of tests including MMPI	9% personality disorder
Robertson (1987)	Winnipeg remand centre, Canada	100 consecutive female arrestees	Clinical interview with a psychologist	Point prevalence of DSM–III antisocial personality disorder 60%
Taylor & Parrott (1988)	Brixton remand prison	23 elderly remand prisoners (>65 years)	Review of prison records using checklist	2/23 had personality disorder
Coid (1988)	Winchester remand prison	334 male remand prisoners	Prison doctor diagnosis from case notes	22/334 had an 'additional diagnosis' of personality disorder
Dell *et al* (1991)	Brixton remand prison	232 male remand prisoners selected for medical report	Clinician's diagnosis	17% psychopathic disorder

contd...

Table 2.8 (*contd...*)

	Setting	Instrument	Sample	Findings
Watt *et al* (1993)	Bristol remand prison	EPQ CAGE BPRS	31 male remand prisoners (20% random sample of new remands)	13% personality disorder
Teplin *et al* (1996)	Cook Co. Department of Corrections, Chicago	DIS	Stratified random sample of 1272 female arrestees awaiting trial	Lifetime prevalence of DSM–III–R antisocial personality disorder 13.8%
Andersen *et al* (1996)	Western prison of Copenhagen	PCL–R Case notes	2 random samples of newly admitted Danish-born prisoners (males & females)	Lifetime prevalence of ICD–10 dissocial personality disorder 17%
Birmingham *et al* (1996)	Durham remand prison	Semi-structured interview (personality disorder diagnosed according to DSM–IV criteria)	569 consecutive male remand prisoners	7% personality disorder In addition, 12% had 'significant personality vulnerabilities'
Maden *et al* (1996)	3 young offenders institutions, 13 adult prisons men's and 3 womens prisons in UK	Semi-structured interview using ICD–10 criteria Case records Interview with prison staff	Stratified random samples of male population (9% total remand population), female (82% total population), and young male offenders (10% total population)	Prevalence personality disorder: males 11.2%; females 15.5%; male youths 11.7%

MMPI, Minnesota Multiphasic Personality Inventory; EPQ, Eysenck Personality Qustionnaire; BPRS, Brief Psychiatric Rating Scale; DIS, Diagnostic Interview Schedule; PCL–R, Psychopathy Checklist, Revised version.

Teplin *et al*, 1996; Andersen *et al*, 1996). The other studies used a variety of different sampling methods and definitions of caseness, making it impossible to come to any conclusions about the prevalence rate of antisocial personality disorder or indeed personality disorder generally in remand prison settings.

The three studies that adopted a more uniform methodology found comparable lifetime prevalence rates of antisocial personality disorder/ personality disorder for both male and female samples. (For females: 13.8% DSM–III–R antisocial personality disorder in Teplin *et al*'s sample compared with 15.5% ICD–10 'personality disorder' in Maden *et al*'s sample; for males: 11% 'personality disorder' in Maden's sample of remanded males and 17% ICD–10 dissocial personality disorder for the predominantly male remand sample in Denmark.)

Teplin *et al* (1996) found that among female jail detainees, the highest prevalence of antisocial personality disorder was in the 18–25 year age group. It also occurred most frequently in White subjects. The authors compared the data with ECA data and established that antisocial personality disorder was 30 times more common among female jail detainees than in female members of the community. This finding was, however, imprecise (95% CI 12.6–73.2) and should be interpreted with the same degree of caution as Jordan's finding in the sentenced female population.

In addition to determining the prevalence of personality disorder in a consecutive remand sample, Birmingham *et al* (1996) also examined the ability of prison reception screening to detect mental disorder. Although the authors did not detail what proportion of disorder remained undetected by the screening process, they concluded that the process is neither sensitive nor specific.

Maden *et al* (1996) used a design similar to that employed by Gunn *et al* (1991) in order to determine the prevalence of mental disorder in cross-sectional samples of remanded men, women and youths. The authors acknowledged that because the assessment procedure for personality disorders was not detailed enough, the prevalence estimates must be regarded as underestimates. Multiple diagnoses were common, with about a third of the total sample receiving two or more diagnoses. Much of this was due to substance misuse. The study looked at the treatment needs of the remand population and found that about half of all subjects suffering from a personality disorder might benefit from treatment and require further assessment for a therapeutic community. It was estimated that, overall, at least 6% of the UK remand population required long-term treatment for personality disorder. On the basis of the survey, the authors made the following recommendations:

(a) There was a need for about 458 places for adult men, 305 for women, and 186 for young offenders, ideally in both the prison system and in the NHS.

(b) In keeping with Jordan's findings in the sentenced female population, about half of the women with a personality disorder were thought to be suffering from borderline personality disorder. In this group, challenging behaviour such as repeated cutting was common, and they proved to be a particularly difficult group to manage. Special facilities were recommended to help develop expertise in meeting the challenges that these women pose to those managing them.

(c) The period of remand should include a thorough assessment, using a variety of standardised diagnostic instruments.

The study's main limitation was its relatively high refusal rate: 19% for men, 10% for young offenders and 6% for women (the more reliable prison surveys have had refusal rates of 5–10%). Both the call-up system employed by the study and the prison regime seemed to influence refusal rates in this study.

Studies in special/high security hospitals

Section 4 of the National Health Service Act 1977 requires the Secretary of State to provide and maintain special hospitals "for persons subject to detention ... who in his opinion require treatment under conditions of special security on account of their dangerous, violent or criminal propensities". For this reason, it is likely that patients in special hospitals will represent the most severely disturbed personalities in clinical practice (Mbatia & Tyrer, 1988). There is, however, little information pertaining to the epidemiology of individual categories of personality disorder in special hospitals.

Using the Personality Assessment Schedule (PAS), Mbatia & Tyrer (1988) estimated the prevalence of categories of personality disorder, including 'sociopathic', in a sample of 103 consecutive admissions to Rampton Hospital. Only patients detained under the legal categories of mental illness and psychopathic disorder were included in the study, and only 30% of these patients had suitable informants available for interview; the remaining interviews relied on self-report. Of the sample (58 patients), 77% were judged to have a personality disorder using a simple classification, and 79% (59 patients) were personality-disordered according to a more detailed procedure. Seventy per cent (41 patients) of those classified as personality-disordered received a PAS diagnosis of sociopathic personality disorder. Of these 41 patients, 11 had received an admission diagnosis of mental illness and 30 had received a diagnosis of personality disorder. A greater proportion of women (82%) had sociopathic personality disorders compared with men (47%), which the authors speculated was probably due to the fact that dangerousness in women is almost always accompanied by sociopathy, whereas in men it can encompass several types of abnormal personality.

Coid (1992) provided epidemiological data on patients detained under the legal category of psychopathic disorder at two maximum security hospitals. A battery of instruments was administered to three subsamples: all males detained under the legal category of psychopathic disorder in Broadmoor Hospital from 1984 to 1986 (n=86); all females detained under the legal category of psychopathic disorder in three maximum security hospitals from 1984 to 1987 (n=93); and, for comparison, disruptive male prisoners in Parkhurst, Lincoln and Hull prisons from 1987 to 1993 (n=64). Lifetime prevalence rates were determined for both axis I and II disorders; axis II disorders were determined using SCID–II. In addition, psychopathy was measured using the PCL–R. Borderline and antisocial personality disorders were the most prevalent disorders, often in combination. Most subjects received multiple axis II diagnoses, with an overall mean of 3.6 (s.d. 1.8; range: 0–9). For borderline disorder, the respective lifetime prevalence rates for female psychopaths, male psychopaths and prisoners were 91, 56 and 55%, respectively. For antisocial personality disorder, the respective rates were 44, 38 and 86%. The proportions of each group that met the PCL–R-defined caseness score for psychopathy were 31, 23 and 77%. It is therefore clear that a substantial proportion of men detained under the legal category of psychopathic disorder in special hospitals were not clinical 'psychopaths', as defined by the Hare construct. This provides further empirical evidence for the disparity between clinical and legal concepts of psychopathy.

In a survey of the treatment and security needs of a stratified random sample of 296 patients from the three special hospitals (20% of all special hospital patients, excluding those who had been in hospital for less than one year), Maden *et al* (1995) found that 24% (n=63) of the sample had a primary diagnosis of ICD–9 personality disorder. Diagnosis was made by the research team on the basis of information collected from hospital case notes, together with semi-structured interviews with the patient and the patient's consultant, although there was no standardised assessment of personality. The authors did not attempt to look at the frequency of categories or clusters of personality disorder, although the survey's primary intention was to examine the service requirements of special hospital patients. Overall, the authors tentatively concluded that the treatment and security needs of patients with personality disorder did not differ markedly from those of other special hospital patients.

As has already been noted, the Mental Health Act 1983 legal category of psychopathic disorder encompasses a wide range of diagnostic categories (Coid, 1992). Furthermore, there will be some who do not have a personality disorder. Nevertheless, in the absence of better epidemiological information on special hospital patients, hospital admission data provide crude estimates of the numbers of patients with antisocial personality disorder referred and admitted to the special hospitals. Based on 1986 figures obtained from all four special hospitals, Hamilton (1990) determined that 24% of all special hospital patients were detained under the category of psychopathic disorder. Of each of the four special hospitals (as they were at the time), the proportions of patients who were detained under the legal category psychopathic disorder were as follows: Broadmoor, 22%; Rampton, 20%; Moss Side, 31%; Park Lane, 26%. Hamilton emphasised that many of the Moss Side and Park Lane psychopaths were of low intelligence.

More recent information on the special hospital patient population comes from the Special Hospitals Service Authority Statistics. Table 2.9 shows the patient population by Mental Health Act 1983 classification and gender, demonstrating the proportion of those who are classified as psychopathically disordered. Table 2.10 shows a breakdown of all referrals and admissions for 1986–1994 by Mental Health Act classification, showing the proportion who are classified

TABLE 2.9

Patient population of special hospitals by Mental Health Act 1983 classification and gender, 1986–1994. (Source: Special Hospitals Service Authority, 1995; reproduced by kind permission of the High Security Psychiatric Services Commissioning Board of the National Health Service Executive)

Year	Mental illness		Psychopathic disorder		Mental impairment		Severe mental impairment	
	Men	Women	Men	Women	Men	Women	Men	Women
1986	851	161	320	93	141	38	44	45
1987	888	161	320	106	131	37	41	40
1988	907	164	321	116	118	36	35	35
1989	910	157	318	109	119	31	34	32
1990	896	151	334	105	108	31	33	31
1991	912	142	341	98	100	31	31	26
1992	943	155	330	88	82	21	31	19
1993	886	156	317	97	75	15	25	15
1994	858	141	310	86	67	11	22	10

TABLE 2.10
*Referrals and admissions to special hospitals by Mental Health Act 1983 classification.
(Source: Special Hospitals Service Authority, 1995; reproduced by kind permission of the
High Security Psychiatric Services Commissioning Board of the National Health Service
Executive)*

Year	Mental illness			Psychopathic disorder			Mental impairment			Severe mental impairment		
	R	A	A/R (%)	R	A	A/R (%)	R	A	A/R (%)	R	A	A/R (%)
1986	177	146	82	98	73	74	36	11	31	4	3	76
1987	201	136	68	93	59	63	37	13	35	6	1	16
1988	192	113	59	83	60	72	38	11	29	3	1	33
1989	176	114	65	84	60	71	36	10	28	6	3	60
1990	165	110	67	92	58	63	28	11	39	2	0	–
1991	165	126	76	107	45	42	24	10	42	0	0	–
1992	198	146	74	109	42	38	21	5	24	0	0	–
1993	238	146	61	144	49	34	12	5	42	0	0	–
1994	265	125	47	131	43	33	0	0	–	0	0	–

R, referral; A, admission; A/R, approximate percentage of referrals gaining admission.

as psychopathically disordered and the proportion of admissions accepted. In total, the special hospitals receive more than 100 referrals each year relating to people with personality disorder, of which between 30 and 60% are accepted. A large proportion of these patients are admitted to special hospitals from the criminal justice system. The figures for psychopathic disorder in Table 2.10 show an increasing number of referrals but a smaller proportion being accepted.

3   Natural history studies

Methodological considerations

The delineation of natural history is one of the major domains for validating a clinical syndrome (Robins & Guze, 1970). Assumptions about the natural history of personality disorders are inherent in their broad description. ICD–10 diagnostic guidelines refer to abnormal behaviour patterns which are "enduring" and which appear during childhood or adolescence and continue into adulthood (World Health Organization, 1992). DSM–IV postulates that personality disorders have an onset which can be traced back to adolescence or early adulthood and are disorders that lead to impairment in social and occupational functioning (American Psychiatric Association, 1994). There is, however, a dearth of empirical research regarding the longitudinal course of personality disorders (Drake & Vaillant, 1988; Perry, 1993; Stone, 1993).

Undoubtedly, the main reason why there exists such a paucity of longitudinal information on personality disorders is that conducting such research is especially problematical. First, the conceptualisation of personality disorder is rapidly evolving, with the result that diagnostic criteria and instrumentation change from one generation to another. Stable case identification is, therefore, difficult to achieve. Second, there are problems in study design. Retrospective studies are dependent upon memories or case records which may not be accurate, whereas although prospective studies circumvent these issues, they force investigators to rely, in a somewhat circular fashion, on outcome variables whose importance is known at the outset of the study.

Many of the natural history studies of antisocial personality disorder rely on recidivism as an outcome measure. In Dolan & Coid's (1993) review of the treatment of antisocial and psychopathic personality disorder, over three-quarters of the reviewed studies used reconviction as the only or main measure of treatment success. They concluded that offending behaviour was not a sufficiently accurate measure of mental state, and rejected the use of such behaviour as a sufficient criterion of outcome. In terms of the accuracy of reconviction as a behavioural index of the outcome of antisocial personality disorder, it is generally agreed that officially recorded crime data grossly underestimate the amount of crime committed. Dolan & Coid (1993) quote a description by Robertson (1989) that describes reconviction as failing "to meet the criteria necessary for scientific evaluation, as it is impossible to obtain sufficient control of the random or error variance contributing to the criterion measure". The same criticisms may be levelled at rehospitalisation or life history measures, such as unemployment, as measures of outcome.

Findings from the literature search

Surprisingly little is known about the natural course and outcome of antisocial personality disorder. Early writers such as Cleckley held that the prognosis was nearly hopeless. Most of what is currently known is based on Robins' pioneering longitudinal study of children referred to a child guidance clinic (Robins, 1966). A detailed account of Robins' findings is beyond the scope of this chapter. In brief, however, the sample comprised 406 White children referred to a child guidance clinic with antisocial behaviour, 118 referred with predominantly neurotic symptoms, and 100 controls recruited from the local neighbourhood. The subjects were followed-up 30 years later. At follow-up interview, of the antisocial group, 75% of men and 40% of women had been arrested for non-traffic offences and almost half the males had been arrested for at least one major crime. Serious offences were only found in the histories of those who had been conduct-disordered children. From these and other findings, Robins devised criteria for the diagnosis of 'sociopathic personality disorder'. At 30-year follow-up, 25% of men and 12% of women were found to meet lifetime criteria for sociopathic personality disorder. In terms of the outcome of sociopathy, Robins judged that at 30 years (when subjects were in their fourth or fifth decade), 12% were in remission, and 27% showed a greatly reduced range in the severity of antisocial behaviour, although 60% still showed little improvement. Most improvement occurred within the 30–40 year age range.

Robins (1978) later replicated her original findings in cohorts of young Black males, Vietnam veterans and matched non-veterans. The following conclusions have been drawn from her studies:

(a) Adult antisocial behaviour virtually requires childhood antisocial behaviour. ECA data (Robins *et al*, 1991) show that looking backwards, 95% of males with four or more adult symptoms had at least one childhood symptom, and 76% had three or more childhood symptoms.

(b) Most antisocial children do not become antisocial adults. (In Robins' study, only 27% of males showing three or more childhood symptoms also showed four or more adult symptoms.)

(c) The variety of antisocial behaviour is a better predictor of adult antisocial behaviour than is any particular behaviour.

(d) Adult antisocial behaviour is better predicted by childhood behaviour than by family background or social class of rearing.

The major studies that have examined the natural course of antisocial personality disorder and which have been published after Robins' original study are listed in Table 3.1. As was previously noted, studies of offending behaviour provide only a very crude measure of the 'outcome' of antisocial personality disorder. Nevertheless, for the sake of completeness, the major studies that have examined reconviction rates in samples of psychopathic patients have also been included. A consistent finding from all of these studies is that a legal classification of psychopathic disorder is a strong correlate of conviction. Taylor (1992) has succinctly remarked that the apparent "glow" of special hospital success in the treatment of the mentally ill is damaged by this high reconviction rate.

Of the 17 studies included, seven are retrospective and 10 prospective in design. The majority of samples are drawn from criminal populations and can be criticised for not being representative of other psychiatric or non-psychiatric populations. Only five of the studies used a standardised diagnostic instrument: the PDQ (further details available from the author upon request) and the PCL (Hart *et al*, 1988; Harris *et al*, 1991; Rice & Harris, 1995; Reiss *et al*, 1996). Four of the remaining studies made an attempt to diagnose antisocial personality disorder using standardised diagnoses: Henderson's criteria (Gibbens *et al*, 1955), Feighner criteria (Guze, 1976) or DSM–III criteria (Martin *et al*, 1982; Arboleda-Florez & Helley, 1991; Black *et al*, 1995*a,b*). Six of the studies rather unsatisfactorily employed only the legal definition of psychopathic disorder, and one study relied entirely on clinical judgement for diagnostic assessment (Maddocks, 1970). Only three of the studies used a control group (Black *et al*, 1995*b*; Rice & Harris 1995; Steels *et al*, 1998). The remaining studies adopted a single group design, making it difficult to determine the discriminant validity of the diagnosis studied.

Length of follow-up in the prospective studies varied from 1.5 years (Hart *et al*, 1988) to 29 years (Black *et al*, 1995*a*). During these follow-up periods, the number of times when data were collected was

TABLE 3.1

Studies of the natural course of psychopathy/antisocial personality disorder

Author	Sample	Diagnosis	Design	Findings
Gibbens et al (1955)	69 'psychopaths' from Wandsworth, Brixton and Wormwood Scrubs + 56 non-psychopathic controls, matched for age and offence	Henderson's criteria	Prospective cohort; single follow-up at 5 years. Follow-up data: criminal records	Proportion 'conviction-free': psychopaths: 12% non-psychopaths: 57%. Offending in psychopathic group diminished with time, although group differences largely accounted for by differences in previous offending history
Maddocks (1970)	59 'psychopaths' recruited from out-patient clinic (= all psychopaths entering clinic over a 3-year period)	Case records (impulsivity taken as core of psychopathy)	Retrospective: single follow-up of 88% of sample at 5.6 years. Follow-up data: case records, clinical interview, informant interview	17% 'settled-down' (reduced impulsivity leading to permanence of employment and a relationship) 66% 'not settled-down' 5% suicide (n=3) 12% lost to follow-up 25% 'chronic alcoholics' 25% 'chronic hypochondriacs'
Acres (1975)	92 patients discharged from the 3 special hospitals during 1971. 47% legally-defined psychopaths (n=43)	MHA classification	Prospective; descriptive study of reconviction rates and after-care, 2 years following discharge	Re-conviction rates per MHA category: subnormality > psychopathy > mental illness
Guze (1976)	223 incarcerated male felons: 79% sociopathy, 54% alcoholism, 5% drug misuse	Feighner's criteria	Prospective; 79% of sample followed over 8–9 years	Of those who were sociopathic at intake, those still sociopathic at 3 years: 87%; 9 years: 72%. 3 violent deaths. High rates of recidivism

contd...

TABLE 3.1 (*contd...*)

Study	Sample	Method	Follow-up	Findings
Martin *et al* (1982)	66 incarcerated female felons. 65% (*n*=43) met DSM–III criteria for antisocial personality disorder. 39 of these qualified for additional diagnoses including alcoholism (47%) and hysteria (41%)	Semi-structured interview using DSM–III criteria	Prospective; sample followed-up at 6 years (99% traced, 66% interviewed)	Criminality: 33% at 3 years; 18% at 6 years. Axis I disorder: somatisation 56%; alcoholism 30%; drug misuse 20%. Psychosocial: 39% received psychiatric treatment at some point; 62% working; 36% married; 1 death by overdose
Tennent & Way (1984)	617 patients discharged from special hospitals. 49% personality-disordered; 33% legally-defined psychopaths (*n*=202)	MHA classification	Prospective; criminal records and case notes examined at 2 follow-ups over a 12 to 17-year period	Psychopaths more likely to commit a violent offence post-release compared with mentally ill
Hart *et al* (1988)	231 men released from prison, 30% high PCL scorers (>34)	22-item PCL	Prospective; high scorers followed for 1.5 years	65% of high PCL–R scorers violated release conditions
Arboleda-Florez & Helley (1991)	38 men, 1 woman with DSM–III antisocial personality disorder, recruited from the forensic unit of a Canadian general hospital	'Clinical diagnosis' using DSM–III antisocial personality disorder criteria	Retrospective; conviction data sought on subjects over 16 to 59-year period	Criminality declined from age 27. Significant proportion remained criminally active
Harris *et al* (1991)	169 mentally disordered offenders recruited from max. security hospital. 31% (*n*=52) psychopaths (all had spent at least 2 years in a therapeutic community programme)	PCL coded retrospectively	Prospective; average length of follow-up: 10 years	Violent recidivism in 77% psychopaths; 21% non-psychopaths

contd...

TABLE 3.1 (*contd...*)

Author	Sample	Diagnosis	Design	Findings
Bailey & MacCulloch (1992)	106 male patients discharged from Park Lane Hospital. 45% legally-defined psychopaths (*n*=50)	MHA classification	Retrospective; hospital and criminal records obtained over an average of 6 years	Psychopaths significantly more likely to be reconvicted compared with mentally ill
Murch & Dolan[1]	142 patients referred to Henderson Hospital, but not admitted. 65% DSM–III–R antisocial personality disorder	PDQ	Prospective audit at 1 year. Referrers contacted for information on psychiatric and forensic status (85% response rate)	68% (*n*=81) seen; 59% (*n*=48) received treatment; 27% (*n*=22) taking psychotropic medication; 17% (*n*=15) convicted of criminal offence; 5% (*n*=4) in prison; 5% (*n*=4) died (3 suicides, 1 killed)
Cope & Ward (1993)	51 special hospital patients admitted to and discharged from medium secure units over a 10-year period. 38% legally-defined psychopaths (*n*=20)	MHA classification	Retrospective case notes study. Mean follow-up period, 5.3 years	Psychopaths more likely to be returned to special hospital (difference was non-significant)
Black *et al* (1995*a,b*)	71 psychiatric in-patients with DSM–III antisocial personality disorder + 225 depressed controls, 200 controls with schizophrenia and 160 surgical controls	Diagnosis assigned retrospectively from case records	Prospective cohort; single follow-up at 29 years. 96% traced, 48% interviewed. Ratings of outcome using GAS	42% unimproved, 31% improved but not remitted, 27% remitted, 22.5% attempted suicide. By comparison with controls: depressed and surgical controls had better GAS ratings in all areas except residential status. Low GAS score at intake associated with poor outcome at follow-up

contd...

TABLE 3.1 (*contd...*)

Rice & Harris (1995)	685 mentally disordered offenders + a group of matched conviction offenders. 22% of study group psychopaths (n=144)	PCL (case notes only)	Prospective cohort; average length of follow-up, 4.5 years	Psychopathy predicted violent recidivism with odds ratio of 3.7 (P < 0.0001)
Reiss *et al* (1996)	49 young males admitted to Broadmoor's Young Person's Unit. Mean PCL–R score: 19.6	Case records used to make DSM–III–R diagnoses, and PCL–R ratings	Retrospective case notes study. Ratings obtained for period of admission (mean length = 4.6 years) and post-discharge	Heterogeneous sample; borderline personality disorder most prevalent. 61% (n=30) eventually discharged to community. Mean length of detention in hospital: 7.8 years. 20% of sample reoffended. 2 deaths (1 suicide, 1 accident)
Buchanan (1998)	All 425 patients discharged from special hospitals in 1982 and 1983. 33% legally-defined psychopaths	MHA classification	Retrospective cohort study. Conviction data sought over 10.5 years post-discharge	Psychopathic disorder predicted conviction greater than mental illness (odds ratio: 2.3; 95% CI 1.4–3.6)
Steels *et al* (1998)	95 patients detained under legal category 'psychopathic disorder'. Control group of 89 detained under 'mental illness' category (93% schizophrenia)	MHA classification	Retrospective; average length of follow-up 14 years. Information sought from case notes. Ratings of outcome using modified Chestnut Lodge outcome scale	No differences in mortality between personality disorder and mental illness groups. Females had more satisfactory outcome irrespective of MHA classification. For male personality disorders, conviction rates x2 and imprisonment rates x4 compared with mental illness, but better psychosocial outcome (x3 working, x4 in a relationship)

PCL, Psychopathy Checklist (PCL–R, Revised version); PDQ, Personality Diagnostic Questionnaire; GAS, Global Assessment Scale.
1. Further details available from the author upon request.

limited, and the vast majority of studies relied entirely upon case records or crime data for outcome information. All of the studies, with the exception of Tennant & Way (1984), collected follow-up data at only one point in time, and none of the studies adopted a design employing multiple follow-ups. Such a design would delineate a more detailed understanding of the course, as opposed to just outcome. (Strauss *et al* (1985) suggested that the longitudinal course of many individuals is not linear, so that one 'snapshot' assessment severely underestimates the true course within individuals.)

An examination of the percentage of each sample followed up indicates that loss of subjects to follow-up is a significant problem. The better rates of follow-up were in the longer-term studies, such as Black *et al* (1995*a,b*), where enough identifying data were available to facilitate subsequent location of the subjects. These findings are consistent with those reporting data on drop-out bias, which indicate that individuals with antisocial personality disorder and males are associated with higher drop-out status.

Finally, the listed studies used a variety of outcome variables. Many of the studies used criminal outcome variables, which are unsatisfactory markers of psychiatric status for the reasons mentioned before. Others have made some attempt to look at broader psychosocial outcome variables, although these are rarely quantified satisfactorily, with the exceptions of Black *et al* (1995*a,b*) who used the Global Assessment Scale, and Steels *et al* (1998) who used outcome dimensions described in the Chestnut Lodge study (McGlashan, 1986).

Undoubtedly the most thoroughly studied axis II disorder, from the longitudinal perspective, has been borderline personality disorder. A number of longitudinal studies of borderline patients have incorporated small groups of antisocial patients in their samples. Perhaps the most important studies falling into this category are the Chestnut Lodge study (McGlashan, 1986) and the PI-500 study (Stone *et al*, 1987). Both studies followed large cohorts of borderline patients for long periods of time (up to 20 years) after an index hospital admission. Both studies confirmed that, generally, the presence of strong antisocial traits predicted a poorer prognosis in borderline personality disorder.

Antisocial 'burn-out'

It has been the popular view of many authors (and clinicians) that antisocial personality disorder 'burns-out' with increasing age, mirroring the postulated decrease in severity with age of personality disorders in general. A variety of views have been expressed on when this will occur; some have suggested between age 25 and the early 30s (Curran & Partridge, 1963) whereas others have suggested the fifth decade (Morris, 1974). Walters (1990) pointed out the important distinction between 'maturity' and 'burn-out'; the former represents a more fundamental psychological shift leading to a redefinition of earlier goals and the abandonment of destructive behaviour, whereas the latter represents the exhaustion of criminal drive by the accumulation of punishments and the ageing process.

The available evidence does not entirely support the burn-out hypothesis, although neither does it entirely refute it. In support of antisocial burn-out, Gibbens *et al* (1955) found that offending in the psychopathic group diminished over time, with 66% of reoffences occurring within one year of release and only 4.3% of offences being committed 3–8 years after release. However, when previous offending histories were taken into account, there were no significant differences between psychopathic and non-psychopathic groups. By looking at diagnostic continuity over time, Guze (1976) was able to demonstrate a reduction in the numbers of subjects rated as sociopathic over time. However, this study used an unsatisfactory, heavily crime-based definition of sociopathy. Martin's group showed a decline in 'criminality' over a six-year follow-up period, although the sample group was heterogeneous and the outcome findings were heavily confounded by state effects. Arboleda-Florez & Helley (1991) demonstrated a decline in offending in a sample of antisocial personalities; the design was, however, retrospective and the sample size too small to draw firm conclusions. Although not strictly speaking a longitudinal study of psychopathy, Harpur & Hare (1994) provided some support for the burn-out hypothesis by showing that PCL subscores decline with age. They assessed 889 male prison inmates between the ages of 16 and 69 with the PCL. Cross-sectional analysis revealed that mean scores on factor 1 (affective–interpersonal traits thought to be central to psychopathy) were stable across the age span, although there was an age-related decline in mean scores on factor 2 (traits and behaviour associated with an unstable lifestyle). The authors acknowledged that alternative explanations other than a maturational effect may explain the findings, such as selection and recall bias.

As evidence against burn-out, Robins judged that only 12% of her subjects were in remission at 30-year follow-up, with 61% showing little improvement. Maddocks (1970) found that the majority of psychopaths had not 'settled down', although this study can be criticised for its retrospective design and its lack of standardised approach to diagnosis. Perhaps the most convincing piece of evidence against antisocial burn-out is Black *et al*'s (1995*a,b*) finding that 42% of a sample of 71 antisocial men were unimproved at 29-year follow-up. Using the Global Assessment Scale, the antisocial subjects were rated as doing significantly worse than the controls with schizophrenia, controls with depression and normal controls on occupational and psychiatric adjustment, although better than the subjects with schizophrenia for marital and residential adjustment. This study is unique in its description of the outcome of antisocial personality disorder in different life domains, yet it too is limited in its method of case identification, single follow-up design and high attrition rate.

Suicide and antisocial personality disorder

Five of the listed studies examined completed suicide as an outcome associated with antisocial personality disorder or psychopathy (Maddocks, 1970; Guze, 1976; Martin *et al*, 1982; Reiss *et al*, 1996; Murch & Dolan, further details available from the author upon request). Estimates vary from 2 to 5% in the studies listed, although the actual numbers of subjects involved are comparatively small. However, none of these studies employed a control group, and therefore no firm conclusions can be drawn about the risk of completed suicide associated with antisocial personality disorder. Lesage *et al* (1994) employed the psychological autopsy method and a case–control design in order to examine the association of specific mental disorders with suicide among a group of young men from Canada. Seventy-five men aged 18–35 years whose deaths received a coroner's verdict of completed suicide were matched to 75 living men for age, place of residence, marital status and occupation. Information was obtained from an interview with a key informant, and coroner and medical records. Two psychiatrists, blind to outcome, then established best-estimate DSM–III–R diagnoses. At least one axis I disorder was identified in 88% of suicide subjects (OR 12.3; 95% CI 5.3–12.5) and at least one axis II disorder was identified in 57% of suicide subjects (OR 4; 95% CI 2–7.9). The commonest axis II disorders were borderline personality disorder (OR 9.3; 95% CI 2.6–33) and antisocial personality disorder (OR 4.1; 95% CI 1–15.4). Using the SAP as part of a biographical reconstructive interview conducted for consecutive suicides from three ethnic groups (two aboriginal groups and a group of Han Chinese in East Taiwan), Cheng *et al* (1997) found that between 47 and 77% of suicide victims suffered from ICD–10 personality disorder. In all groups, the most prevalent category among suicides was emotionally unstable personality disorder, occurring in 41% of suicides (OR 9.9; 95% CI 4.6–21.1). Dissocial personality disorder was identified in only 3.5% of suicides.

While there remains a lack of consensus (based on a paucity of robust research) on whether individuals with antisocial personalities are at higher risk of completed suicide, the literature indicates that there is an association with attempted suicide. Early research in this area indicated a strong association, although it was methodologically flawed. For example, Woodruff *et al* (1971) reported suicide attempts in 23% of antisocial subjects, although the findings were limited by the small sample size (*n*=35). More recently, Garvey & Spoden (1980) estimated that 72% of a sample of 39 mental health centre attenders diagnosed with antisocial personality disorder had made a total of 63 previous suicide attempts. Again, this study's findings are limited by the highly selected nature and small size of the sample involved.

Better data on the association between antisocial personality disorder and suicide attempts come from Dyck *et al* (1988) and Beautrais *et al* (1996). Dyck *et al* (1988) examined the lifetime histories of attempted suicide and psychiatric disorders (using the DIS) on a random sample of 3258 household residents of Edmonton, Canada. By comparing the prevalence of psychiatric disorder in attempters and non-attempters, they were able to calculate the relative risk of attempted suicide for each disorder. Approximately 80% of those with a history of suicide attempts had a lifetime psychiatric disorder. The greatest relative risks were associated with schizophrenia (23.1) and mania (21.0). The relative risk for antisocial personality disorder was 4.0.

Beautrais *et al* (1996) adopted a case–control design in order to test the association between mental disorders and attempted suicide; 302 consecutive subjects who made serious suicide attempts were compared with 1028 randomly-selected controls. Each subject was interviewed with a modified version of the Structured Clinical Interview for DSM–III–R disorders. Of those who attempted suicide, 90.1% had a mental disorder at the time of the attempt. Multiple logistic regression was performed on the data, in order to take account of comorbidity of different mental disorders. This showed that the odds of a serious suicide attempt were significantly higher for individuals with a diagnosis of mood disorder (OR 33.4; 95% CI 21.9–51.2), substance use disorder (OR 2.6; 95% CI 1.6–4.3) or antisocial personality disorder (OR 3.7; 95% CI 2.1–6.5). However, an estimation of the population-attributable risk showed that only elimination of mood disorders would result in a substantial reduction in the frequency of attempted suicide.

In keeping with the literature on the association between suicidal behaviour and antisocial personality disorder are findings from prospective and retrospective studies that a diagnosis of antisocial personality disorder is highly predictive of death from unnatural causes. In a 6 to 12-year follow-up of 500 psychiatric out-patients, Martin *et al* (1985) found that a diagnosis of antisocial personality disorder was associated with a significant excess of unnatural causes of death (largely suicide, accidents and homicides). In the reference population, the standardised mortality ratio for unnatural deaths was 4.3. The standardised mortality ratios for antisocial personality disorder and drug disorders were both significantly in excess of this, with rates of 14.7 and 16.7 respectively. Retrospective data confirm that antisocial personality disorder is a risk factor for both sudden violent death (Rydelius, 1988) and accidental injury (McDonald & Davey, 1996).

Conclusions from longitudinal studies

In the light of the aforementioned criticisms, it is difficult to come to any firm conclusions about the natural course of antisocial personality disorder. However, certain trends do emerge from the data. The better data that examine psychosocial outcome variables suggest that antisocial personality disorder is a chronic disorder associated with ongoing psychiatric, medical and social problems, a finding which is perhaps not wholly unexpected given the impulsive and destructive nature of this group. Epidemiological data also suggest that antisocial personality disorder is associated with attempted suicide, although perhaps not as strongly as was once thought. Antisocial burn-out remains neither wholly supported nor refuted as a theory. What is less clear from the research is the nature of the mechanism that lies behind adverse outcome, and what protective factors are associated with a 'better' outcome. Put differently, why do some individuals with antisocial personality disorder or 'psychopathic traits' go on to pursue an irrevocably destructive life history, while others live a more quiescent or even successful existence (Hart & Hare, 1994; Babiak, 1995)?

4 Studies of associated conditions

This chapter provides a review of the various personality disorders and mental illnesses associated with antisocial personality disorder and its diagnostic equivalents. There is a large international literature on this subject, and it is unfortunately not possible to cover all the relevant published literature comprehensively within this chapter. Instead, an overview of the subject will be presented.

The co-occurrence of independent psychiatric disorders in an individual is often referred to as 'comorbidity'. Possibly the clearest description of this phenomenon has been provided by Feinstein (1970), who defines comorbidity as "any distinct additional clinical entity that has existed or that may occur during the clinical course of a patient who has the index disease under study". There is, however, confusion in the contemporary epidemiological literature as to the appropriate use of the term. Currently, the term is often used to mean the simultaneous presence of two or more DSM–IV disorders. The disorders may arise from the same axis as well as from different axes. Tyrer (1996) has highlighted the issue central to the conceptual confusion surrounding comorbidity research:

> "The major problem is that what is true comorbidity (separate diseases) and what is false comorbidity (consanguinity, or such an intimate relationship between the disorders that they are one and the same) is difficult to determine."

Variability in the definitions and assessments of comorbidity used in studies has led to an increasingly complex and confusing picture of the concept. These factors have led to substantial variation in the magnitude of estimated comorbidity across studies (Wittchen, 1996). In the field of the personality disorders, many of the axis II comorbidity studies overestimate the level of true comorbidity. Explanations for this include the artefactual comorbidity that occurs due to overlapping diagnostic criteria, the tendency for some instruments (particularly self-report instruments) to overdiagnose personality disorders, and the failure of most studies to control for confounding from multiple diagnostic covariation in the statistical analysis (Coid, 1996).

In the light of these factors, and by way of an attempt to preserve simplicity, the term comorbidity will not be used. Instead, an overview of the literature on those axis I and axis II disorders which have been shown to be associated with antisocial personality disorder will be presented.

Axis II conditions

Research in psychiatric settings suggests that many individuals fulfil criteria for more than one of the personality disorder categories (Morey, 1988). Studies using standardised instruments have demonstrated that at least 50% of subjects can be expected to have two or more coexisting personality disorders (Pfohl *et al*, 1986; Loranger *et al*, 1987; Oldham *et al*, 1992). This is perhaps an inevitable result of the application of the categorical approach to the assessment of personality and has led to justifiable criticism of this approach (Vize & Tyrer, 1994). In addition, some of the instruments available for assessing personality disorders, notably self-report instruments such as the PDQ, have a very low threshold for diagnosing personality disorders and consequently generate a significant number of 'false positives'. For example, Dolan *et al* (1995) used the PDQ–R to assess personality disorders in three UK samples: referrals for specialist in-patient treatment ($n = 275$), high tariff offenders ($n=57$), and undergraduate students ($n=274$). The mean numbers of axis II disorders per subject were 6.0 (95% CI 5.7–6.3), 4.0 (95% CI 3.1–5.0) and 3.4 (95% CI 3.0–3.8) respectively. Clearly a finding of six personality disorders per subject is clinically meaningless, although the authors discuss the possibility of such a finding forming a crude measure of the range of disturbance.

Coid (1996) has reviewed the published literature on intra-axis II co-occurrence. Only studies that employed a standardised assessment procedure to establish axis II diagnoses (or dimensional scores) were included. Studies that used self-report data were excluded because of the tendency to overdiagnose personality disorders by this method. Coid's data on antisocial personality disorder are presented in Table 4.1. The table has three components: correlation coefficients between dimensional scores derived from research interview schedules; Widiger's calculations for the average of correlations of personality disorder across nine studies; and finally categorical data (presented as odds ratios) from a study published by Oldham *et al* (1992). It is important to note that none of the studies controlled

TABLE 4.1

Covariation of antisocial personality disorder with other personality disorders (adapted from Coid, 1996, by kind permission of the author)

Study	Method	Sample	Number with antisocial personality disorder	PARA	ZOID	SZTP	HIST	NAR	BOR	AVOI	DEPT	COM	PAG
Interview dimensional													
Hyler & Lyons (1988)	Clinician	358	8	0.22	0.17	0.09	0.22	0.40	0.29	0.02	0.10	-0.03	0.28
Kass *et al* (1985)	Clinician	609	12	0.10	0.14	0.04	0.11	0.20	0.26	0.02	-0.08	-0.10	0.04
Widiger *et al* (1987)	Clinician	84	31	0.31	0.06	0.15	0.33	0.22	0.43	0.14	0.00	0.18	0.31
Samuels *et al* (1994)	Clinician	95	20	0.30	0.04	-0.04	0.33	0.23	0.37	0.01	-0.02	0.02	0.12
Zimmerman & Coryell (1989)	SIDP	143	26	0.33	0.12	0.18	0.36	0.48	0.54	0.16	0.07	0.23	0.26
Moldin *et al* (1994)	PDE	302	8	0.28	0.04	0.34	0.36	0.50	0.68	0.28	0.27	0.20	0.29
Average				0.26	0.10	0.14	0.29	0.34	0.43	0.11	0.06	0.08	0.22
Average across 9 studies													
Widiger *et al* (1991)				0.23	0.12	0.15	0.24	0.33	0.37	0.03	0.07	-0.02	0.35
Interview categorical													
Oldham *et al* (1995)	SCID	100	7	2.7	1.2	0.7	4.6	8.2	10.4	0.7	0.3	1.9	6.2
	PDE	100	9	1.7	3.2	2.3	14.5	6.3	1.1	0.4	2.7	0.4	1.5

PARA, paranoid; ZOID, schizoid; SZTP, schizotypal; HIST, histrionic; NAR, narcissistic; BOR, borderline; AVOI, avoidant; DEPT, dependent; COM, compulsive; PAG, passibe-aggressive; SIDP, Structured Interview for DSM–III Personality Disorders; PDE, Personality Disorder Examination; SCID, Structured Clinical Interview for DSM–III Personality Disorders.

for state-dependent ratings. All data were derived from samples of psychiatric patients, with the exception of the data from studies by Moldin and Samuels, both of whom used community samples.

From the table, it can be seen that antisocial personality disorder consistently demonstrates a high level of covariation with histrionic, narcissistic and borderline personality disorders. Coid (1996) suggested that the relatively high odds ratios found with schizoid, schizotypal and dependent personality disorders should probably be discounted, as they are not confirmed by the meta-analysis, dimensional scores, or SCID.

In Coid's own study of the covariation of axis II disorders in three groups of antisocial subjects, following logistic regression analysis, statistically significant adjusted odds ratios were found between antisocial personality disorder and the following personality disorders: borderline (OR 2.0; 95% CI 1.7–3.5), narcissistic (OR 2.4; 95% CI 1.5–4.1), paranoid (OR 4.5; 95% CI 2.7–7.7), passive–aggressive (OR 2.5; 95% CI 1.3–4.6). The high covariation with paranoid disorder has not been found in other studies, and Coid suggested that the finding may reflect the nature and severity of psychopathology in the sample (Coid, 1996). The other unexpected finding from this study was the absence of an association between antisocial personality disorder and histrionic personality disorder. Logistic regression analysis revealed that an initial association with histrionic disorder was due to confounding by mutually covarying narcissistic and passive–aggressive personality disorders.

Axis I conditions

The establishment of the multiaxial approach to classification as enshrined in DSM–III has been followed by a burgeoning amount of research into the relationship between mental state and personality disorders. The importance in achieving a better understanding of this relationship is highlighted by the fact that the presence of personality pathology in patients with axis I disorders has important clinical implications, especially for predicting poorer response to treatment (Reich & Vasile, 1993).

The nature of the relationship is complex. Some authors have drawn attention to the similarities between the features and supposed aetiologies of certain personality disorders and clinical syndromes, and raised the possibility that the former may be subclinical or even atypical manifestations of the latter (Paris, 1992). Others have considered the possibility of personality disorders acting as vulnerability factors for mental illness (Clarkin & Kendall, 1992). Siever & Davis (1991) have proposed a psychobiological model of personality disorders that postulates cluster-specific axis I–axis II relationships with biological bases. They propose that at the core of antisocial and borderline personality disorders is a psychobiological dimension of impulsivity/aggression. It is postulated that this dimension is shared with axis I impulse disorders.

The assessment of the relationship between personality disorders and mental illness is complicated by two main factors: the contamination of personality assessment by the concurrent presence of mental illness, and the aetiological issues of personality change both preceding and following mental illness. The importance of state bias in the assessment of personality disorders has been consistently demonstrated by a number of studies (e.g. Reich & Noyes, 1987). Loranger *et al* (1991) have, however, shown that a carefully executed interview can yield accurate personality disorder diagnoses in spite of a current axis I state. (The importance of the process of personality change in association with mental illness has been given official recognition in ICD–10, which includes a specific diagnostic code (F62.1) for "enduring personality change after psychiatric illness".)

Methods adopted for examining inter-axis associations have varied considerably, making it difficult to draw comparisons between findings. Three groups of studies may be identified: those that examine the full range of disorders from both axes and then carry out a statistical examination of associations between the individual categories; those that examine clusters of personality disorder and/ or broad groupings of clinical syndromes and then carry out a statistical examination of associations; and, finally, those that select a single axis I category and examine the full range of axis II disorders, or alternatively select a single axis II category (for the purposes of this review, antisocial personality disorder) and examine a range of axis I disorders. Each of these study designs will now be considered.

Studies examining the full range of axis I and axis II disorders

This type of study undoubtedly provides the most complete data on associations between individual axis I and II disorders. Unfortunately, such data are rare; only two studies were identified adopting this approach: Alnæs & Torgesen (1988) and Zimmerman & Coryell (1989). The former study failed to identify any cases of antisocial personality disorder, largely because of the exclusion of patients with substance misuse. Zimmerman & Coryell (1989) interviewed 797 first-degree relatives of patients with psychiatric disorder and normal controls, with standardised instruments, in order to establish the lifetime prevalence and degree of covariation of axis I and II disorders in a high-risk, non-patient sample. State effects were not controlled for in the assessment of personality status. The lifetime prevalences of axis I disorders in 26 subjects with antisocial personality disorder (3.3% of total sample – the most prevalent personality disorder found) were: mania 11.5%; major depression 34.6%; dysthymia 7.7%; alcohol misuse/dependence 76.9%*; drug misuse/dependence 53.8%*; schizophrenia 3.8%; obsessive–compulsive disorder 3.8%; phobic disorder 26.9%; panic disorder 7.7%; bulimia 0%; tobacco use disorder 69.2%*; psychosexual dysfunction 38.5%; lifetime history of attempted suicide 15.4%. (NB. For those disorders marked *, the difference between antisocial personality disorder and individuals with all other personality disorders was significant at the 0.001 level.)

Studies examining clusters of axis II disorders and/or groups of clinical syndromes

Four studies using this design were identified, and their main findings with respect to antisocial personality disorder or cluster B disorders are given in Table 4.2. Jackson *et al* (1991) is the only study of this type that properly controlled for state effects by quantitatively assessing affective symptoms and negative symptoms of schizophrenia. However, the authors acknowledged that the small numbers involved in each group may have explained the failure of this study to demonstrate some significant axis I–axis II associations.

The studies by Maier *et al* (1992) and Nestadt *et al* (1992) have the advantage of looking for axis I–II associations in community groups, and, compared with psychiatric samples, are less likely to have produced spurious associations due to selection bias. Maier *et al* found a strong association between cluster B disorders and affective disorders; however, the extremely low frequency of antisocial personality disorder in this study (one case among 452 subjects, 0.2%) limited any specific conclusions about this disorder. Nestadt *et al* used a two-stage population survey to assess axis I–II associations. A dimensional scoring system based on DSM–III was used to identify antisocial subjects. Subjects who met DSM–III criteria for a diagnosis of antisocial personality disorder (1.5% of the population) were at the extreme of the antisocial scale distribution. Using logistic regression to control for confounding (the only study in this group to use this type of analysis), the authors found that increasing scores on the antisocial personality scale were associated with smaller odds of generalised anxiety disorder and significantly greater odds of alcohol use disorder.

Finally, Oldham *et al* (1995) used standardised instruments to assess associations in a mixed population of 100 long-term applicants for in-patient treatment of personality psychopathology and 100 applicants for psychoanalysis. State effects were not controlled for.

Three per cent of the total sample ($n=7$) were diagnosed with antisocial personality disorder, and odds ratios (95% CIs) for the co-occurrence of axis I disorders and antisocial personality disorder were: mood disorder: 0.5 (0.1–2.5); anxiety disorder: 1.2 (0.3–5.4); psychotic disorder: 2.0 (0.2–17.5); substance use disorder: 1.1 (0.1–9.2) and eating disorder: 1.4 (0.2–12.6). The wide confidence intervals suggest imprecise odds ratio estimates for psychosis and eating disorders, and the failure to find a significant association between antisocial personality disorder and substance use disorder (a finding in virtually all other studies) is possibly attributable to a type 2 error (i.e. the small numbers of antisocial patients in this study).

Studies examining specific categories of axis I disorder

This is the least satisfactory method for determining inter-axis associations, since few axis I disorders occur in isolation over the

TABLE 4.2
Studies examining the association between antisocial personality disorder/cluster B disorders and groups of axis I disorders

Study	Sample	Instruments	Findings
Jackson *et al* (1991)	112 psychiatric in-patients: schizophrenia=35; mania=26; unipolar=30; 'mixed'=21	SIDP; SCID–P; state effects controlled for using: BDI, SANS, MRS	67% had 1 plus personality disorder Frequency of antisocial personality disorder: schizophrenia 20% ($n=7$) mania 15% ($n=4$)
Maier *et al* (1992)	452 community residents	SADS–L, SCID–II	*Prev. any personality disorder:* males: 9.6%; females: 10.3% *Of those with cluster B disorder:* 33% major depression 44% other affective disorder 11% anxiety disorder
Nestadt *et al* (1992)	810 community residents	Dimensional scoring system based on DSM–III	1.5% met caseness for antisocial personality disorder Increasing scores on antisocial scale associated with increased odds of alcohol use disorder
Oldham *et al* (1995)	200 in-patients and out-patients	SCID–P; SCID–II; PDE	3.5% had antisocial personality disorder. Increased odds ratios for disorders: psychosis, eating, substance use, anxiety

SIDP, Structured Interview for DSM–III Personality Disorders; SCID–II, Structured Clinical Interview for DSM–III Personality Disorders; SCID–P, Structured Clinical Interview for DSM–III–R, Patient Version; BDI, Beck Depression Inventory; SANS, Scale for the Assessment of Negative Symptoms; MRS, Mania Rating Scale; SADS–L, Schedule for Affective Disorders and Schizophrenia, Lifetime version; PDE, Personality Disorder Examination.

lifespan of a single subject, and spurious associations may arise due to the presence of additional but unreported axis I disorders (Coid, 1996). Nevertheless, these studies are easier to carry out, and consequently there is an enormous amount of this type of literature.

Substance use disorders

The most heavily studied associated conditions have been substance use disorders. Research at all epidemiological levels confirms a strong association with antisocial personality disorder, and highlights the implications in terms of poorer treatment outcome (e.g. Woody *et al*, 1985; Rounsaville *et al*, 1986). However, the nature of the relationship is complex and, before discussing the main findings from different levels of care, consideration needs to be given to some of the methodological and theoretical issues that underpin this area of research.

The high frequency of antisocial personality disorder in samples of alcohol and other substance misusers has raised quesions about the validity and usefulness of the distinction between substance use disorders and antisocial personality disorder. In DSM–I, alcoholism and other drug addictions were classified as personality disorders and regarded as specific subtypes of sociopathic personality disturbance. In DSM–II, they were no longer classified as personality disorders but, together with sexual deviations, were grouped under the heading of personality disorders and certain other non-psychotic mental disorders. In DSM–III and IV, substance use disorders are clearly separated from personality disorders, and appear on different axes; however, many of the diagnostic criteria overlap. For example, one of the criteria for substance use disorder in DSM–IV is "recurrent substance-related legal problems". Such diagnostic overlap may artificially increase rates of antisocial personality disorder among substance misusers. Despite such diagnostic overlap, longitudinal studies suggest that, at least for alcoholism and antisocial personality disorder, the aetiological factors are different (Cadoret *et al*, 1985).

Clinically, it is often extremely difficult to separate the chronic behavioural disorder associated with drug addiction from the longer-term behaviours or traits associated with personality disorders. Khantzian & Treece (1985) stated that substance use disorder and personality disorders are inextricably intertwined, with each affecting the other in turn. These authors viewed difficulties with dysphoric affect as a central causative feature of both substance use and personality disorder. A further underlying problem is the establishment of the temporal sequence between mental disorders (in this case, antisocial personality disorder) and substance misuse. Put simply, one of two mechanisms may be invoked:

(a) antisocial personality disorder predisposes to substance misuse, *or*

(b) substance misuse predisposes to antisocial personality disorder.

As to which of these is in operation in individuals with both disorders is unclear, although evidence from the National Comorbidity Survey (Kessler *et al*, 1996) favours the former mechanism.

At the community level, representative data on the association between antisocial personality disorder and substance misuse come from the ECA study and the National Comorbidity Survey. Regier *et al* (1990) estimated the lifetime prevalence of comorbid alcohol, other drug, and other mental disorders in a US community population of 20 291 subjects, as part of the ECA programme. Lifetime prevalence rates for mental disorders were determined using the DIS. Estimated lifetime prevalence rates (after logistic regression) were 13.5% for alcohol dependence/misuse and 6.1% for other drug dependence/misuse. The prevalence of antisocial personality disorder among those subjects with an alcohol disorder was 14.3% (adjusted odds ratio 21). The prevalence of antisocial personality disorder among those with any other drug disorder was 17.8% (adjusted odds ratio 13.4). The odds ratios obtained were higher than for any other disorder. Data from the combined prison sample showed that, of those prisoners with antisocial personality disorder (33% of the prison sample), 90% had a comorbid addictive disorder (adjusted odds ratio 5.2).

The National Comorbidity Survey (Kessler *et al*, 1996) provided the first nationally representative data on psychiatric disorder and comorbidity. Lifetime co-occurrence was examined for antisocial personality disorder and also conduct disorder. For antisocial personality disorder, lifetime co-occurrences (presented as odds ratios) were: alcohol dependence, 10.5; drug dependence, 13.6; and misuse/dependence on alcohol and/or drugs, 11.8. In total, almost 80% of all respondents with antisocial personality disorder also had a lifetime addiction disorder. In over 90% of cases, the conduct disorder or antisocial personality disorder preceded the addictive disorder. Antisocial personality disorder was one of only two disorders shown to predict significantly the course of alcohol dependence (the other disorder was primary anxiety disorder).

There are major methodological limitations associated with both the ECA study and the National Comorbidity Survey. Both were cross-sectional surveys that relied entirely on retrospective reports to assess the lifetime prevalence of disorder. In addition, diagnostic assessments were based on only a single interview, administered by a non-clinician. Both factors result in reduced diagnostic precision, and the authors emphasise that the figures should be interpreted cautiously.

TABLE 4.3
Studies of the frequency of antisocial personality disorder (DSM–III unless otherwise stated) in samples of opiate addicts

Study	Sample	Instrument	Prevalence
Kosten *et al* (1982)	384 in-patient/out-patient opiate addicts	Clinical interview	55%
Khantzian & Treece (1985)	133 in-patient/out-patient/ untreated opiate addicts	Clinical interview	35%
Zimmerman & Coryell (1989)	60 opiate addicts	SIDP	23%
Kleinman *et al* (1990)	776 out-patient opiate addicts	Clinical interview	21%
Nace *et al* (1991)	100 in-patient opiate addicts	SCID–II	3%
Dinwiddie *et al* (1992)	(a) 92 i.v. drug-users (b) 230 other drugs (c) 329 cannabis-users (d) 411 non-drug-users	HELPER interview	Antisocial personality disorder (Feighner criteria) (a) 69%; (b) 35%; (c) 21%; (d) 6%;
Gill *et al* (1992)	55 methadone maintenance clients	DIS	42%
Brooner *et al* (1993)	272 i.v. drug-users	DIS	44%
DeJong *et al* (1993)	86 opiate addicts	SIDP	48%
Darke *et al* (1994)	222 methadone maintenance clients	DIS	61%
Kokkevi & Stefanis (1995)	176 opiate addicts mixed in-patient/prisoner group	DIS	69%
Brooner *et al* (1997)	716 out-patient opiate addicts stabilised on methadone for 4–5 weeks	SCID NEO–PI	25.1% (DSM–III–R) (m>f). Rate of antisocial personality disorder equalled that of all non-substance axis I diagnoses combined

SIDP, Structured Interview for DSM–III Personality Disorders; SCID–II, Structured Clinical Interview for DSM–III Personality Disorders; i.v., intravenous; HELPER, Home Environment and Lifetime Psychiatric Evaluation Record; DIS, Diagnostic Interview Schedule; NEO, NEO Personality Inventory.

TABLE 4.4

Studies of the frequency of antisocial personality disorder (DSM–III unless otherwise stated) in samples of cocaine addicts, solvent misusers and people with alcoholism

Study	Sample	Instrument	Prevalence
Cocaine addicts			
Weiss & Mirin (1986)	30 in-patients	Structured clinical interview	3%
Kleinman *et al* (1990)	76 out-patients	SCID–II	21%
Rounsaville *et al* (1991)	298 in-patients + out-patients	SADS–L	RDC antisocial personality disorder 7.7%
Carroll *et al* (1993)	399 in-patients + out-patients	SADS–L	RDC antisocial personality disorder 29%
Weiss *et al* (1993)	50 in-patients	Modified SCID–II	22%
Kranzler *et al* (1994)	50 in-patients	SCID–II	28%
Barber *et al* (1996)	289 out-patients	SCID–II	19.7%
Alcohol misusers			
DeJong *et al* (1993)	178 in-patients	SIDP	5%
Tomasson & Vaglum (1995)	351 in-patients	DIS	28%: m=33%; f=9%
Ross (1995)	8116 household residents: 6% alcohol dependent; 6% alcohol misuse	CIDI (revised)	Of alcohol dependent, 12% antisocial personality disorder
Solvent misusers			
Dinwiddie *et al* (1990)	(a) 130 solvent misusers (b) 2013 non-users	HELPER	Antisocial personality disorder (Feighner criteria) (a) 63%; (b) 12%

SCID–II, Structured Clinical Interview for DSM–III Personality Disorders; SADS–L, Schedule for Affective Disorders and Schizophrenia, Lifetime version; SIDP, Structured Interview for DSM–III Personality Disorders; DIS, Diagnostic Interview Schedule; CIDI, Composite International Diagnostic Interview; HELPER, Home Environment and Lifetime Psychiatric Evaluation Record.

The main studies that have examined the association between antisocial personality disorder and substance misuse in populations of substance users are listed in Tables 4.3 and 4.4. Studies not using standardised diagnoses were excluded. The majority of studies have examined prevalence of DSM–III antisocial personality disorder, although some of the studies have used RDC or Feighner's criteria. The studies generally indicate that opiate dependency has higher levels of co-occurrence with antisocial personality disorder than other disorders, with estimates of between 40 and 60% in some of the studies. Unfortunately, much of the consistency of this research is undermined by the aforementioned methodological problems. In addition, the instrumentation, diagnostic criteria used, and populations sampled vary considerably between studies, hence the wide range of estimates. Very few studies have controlled for state effects in the assessment of antisocial personality disorder. Those studies which have compared diagnoses at a time of dependence on a substance with lifetime diagnoses suggested that this is an important factor. For example, in a 2.5-year follow-up study of 200 opioid addicts, Rounsaville & Kleber (1985) found that half of those with an original diagnosis of antisocial personality disorder were no longer diagnosed with antisocial personality disorder at follow-up.

An important finding from some of the research into opiate addiction is the association between antisocial personality disorder, HIV risk-taking behaviour and HIV status. Gill *et al* (1992) interviewed 55 consecutive methadone maintenance out-patients with the DIS and an HIV risk behaviour interview. Intravenous drug-use was significantly more frequent in the antisocial personality disorder group, as was needle-sharing and the number of needle-sharing partners. On the other hand, using a similar methodology, Darke *et al* (1994) were unable to replicate these findings. Dinwiddie *et al* (1992) found that any history of injecting drugs increased the odds of being diagnosed with antisocial personality disorder by a factor of 21, alcoholism by 4.4 and unipolar depression by 3. A diagnosis of antisocial personality disorder increased the odds of having injected drugs by a factor of 27.2, while diagnoses of alcoholism or unipolar depression conveyed odds for injecting drugs of 4.6 and 3.7 respectively. Brooner *et al* (1993) examined the relationship between a diagnosis of antisocial personality disorder and HIV infection; 272 mainly Black intravenous drug-users (52% of whom were in methadone treatment) were interviewed with the DIS and an HIV risk behaviour interview, before being given an HIV blood test. After controlling for ethnicity, gender, and current methadone treatment status, the diagnosis of antisocial personality disorder was associated with a significantly higher infection rate (uniform odds ratio = 2.44; 95% CI 1.06–5.49). Significant differences were found between those subjects with and those without antisocial personality disorder in the median number of drug injections, the median number of needle-sharing occasions, and the percentage reporting multiple needle-sharing partners for the past year and five-year average. In all cases, the direction of the difference was towards more risk of HIV exposure in those with antisocial personality disorder. The authors concluded that the association is probably due to the poor impulse control and low harm-avoidance characteristic of antisocial personality disorder. Unfortunately, the strength of the association found in this study is undermined by the failure to control for possible confounding effects from the spectrum of drug use and sexual practices, both of which could explain the findings. Clearly more research is required in order to clarify the nature of this relationship.

Finally, research in a variety of forensic settings confirms the high degree of association between antisocial personality disorder and drug disorders. Virtually all the studies of remand and sentenced populations (listed in Tables 2.7 and 2.8) have found a high degree of association. For example, Côté & Hodgins (1990) found that in their random sample of 650 penitentiary inmates the combination of antisocial personality disorder plus alcohol misuse/dependence plus drug misuse/dependence was the most common pattern of co-occurring disorder.

The specific association between psychopathy and substance use disorders has been explored by some studies. Smith & Newman (1990) assessed 360 sentenced prisoners with the PCL and the DIS. Subjects were trichotomised into 'high scorers'/psychopaths (PCL score > 30; 31% of sample), middle scorers (34%) and controls (34%). An increasing gradient in the proportion of alcohol and drug diagnoses was found from control to middle to psychopathic subjects. The odds ratio for co-occurring psychopathy and alcohol misuse/dependence was 5.1 ($P < 0.01$), and for psychopathy and any drug dependence was 2.7 ($P < 0.01$). In addition, the number of DIS alcohol symptoms correlated significantly with the total PCL factor 2 score.

In a meta-analysis of four studies that had examined the relationship between psychopathy and drug misuse/dependence in forensic samples, Hemphill *et al* (1994) found a "consistent and moderate association" between the two types of disorder. Finally, in his study of the psychopathology of legally defined psychopaths and dangerous prisoners, Coid (1996) found that antisocial personality disorder had the highest prevalence in subjects with substance use disorder. Over two-thirds of subjects with both alcoholism and drug dependence/misuse received a diagnosis of antisocial personality disorder.

Other axis I disorders

The National Comorbidity Survey has shown that co-occurrence of multiple psychiatric conditions is the rule rather than the exception.

Kessler *et al* (1994) have shown that, at least in the US, morbidity is highly concentrated – the majority of lifetime disorders occur in roughly one-sixth of the population who experience a lifetime history of three or more disorders. It should therefore come as no surprise to find that antisocial personality disorder has been shown to covary with most axis I conditions, although the degree of covariation is much less than that found in association with substance use disorders. It is beyond the scope of this chapter to present data on all axis I disorders; suffice to say, significant covariation with antisocial personality disorder has been reported in samples of subjects with the following disorders: depression (e.g. Sanderson *et al*, 1992; Pepper *et al*, 1995), phobic disorders (e.g. Renneberg *et al*, 1992), panic and anxiety disorders (e.g. Hoffart *et al*, 1994), eating disorders (e.g. Braun *et al*, 1994), schizophrenia (e.g. Bland *et al*, 1987), obsessive–compulsive disorder (Kolada *et al*, 1994) and pathological gambling (e.g. Bland *et al*, 1993). Few of these studies control for state effects in the assessment of personality, and findings have not been consistently replicated for any of these disorders.

Conclusions

In summary, recent epidemiological research has shown that co-occurrence of mental disorder is extremely common. Antisocial personality disorder behaves like other conditions in this respect, although the accurate assessment of covariation with other axis II disorders and axis I disorders is complicated by the shortcomings of the current categorical classification system, poor specificity of some of the personality assessment instruments used, and a number of confounding factors, the most important of which are state effects. Few studies have assessed the full range of axis I and axis II disorders, and the majority of the studies have focused on specific categories of axis I disorder – data from which give an inaccurate impression of which conditions are most likely to occur in association with antisocial personality disorder. Nevertheless, robust axis II associations have been found with other cluster B disorders and with substance use disorders. The significance of these findings lies in the fact that a large body of research has shown that the management of a range of psychiatric illness is complicated by the presence of an axis II disorder. In terms of recommendations for future research, ultimately the best method of assessing the predisposition of antisocial personality disorder to specific axis I and II disorders would be to follow up high-risk populations over a considerable period of time. As we shall see, such populations could include conduct-disordered children, or antisocial adolescents. By using repeated measures over time, it should be possible to determine which subjects develop antisocial personality disorder, and whether some antisocial subjects develop specific axis I and axis II conditions.

5 Studies of risk factors

It is beyond the scope of this book to give a comprehensive account of the literature on risk factors associated with antisocial personality disorder. For a detailed account, the reader is referred to one of the more extensive reviews on the subject (e.g. Loeber, 1982; Wolff, 1993). The aim of this chapter is to provide an overview of the main findings from risk factor studies and to highlight some of the more important recent developments in this area. The literature falls into one of two major categories: genetic studies that examine the heritability of antisocial personality disorder, and studies of the childhood antecedents of antisocial personality disorder. Each of these categories will now be considered.

Genetic studies of antisocial personality disorder

Genetic studies have examined the following constructs: juvenile delinquency, conduct disorder, adult criminality, antisocial personality disorder and substance misuse. The nature of the genetic relationship between these constructs is uncertain, and the results from some studies may not apply entirely to antisocial personality disorder (Coid, 1996).

Family studies

In one of the first family studies of convicted felons, Guze *et al* (1967) found elevated rates of hysteria, sociopathy, alcoholism and drug addiction among first-degree relatives. Further studies by the same group noted an increased rate of psychopathy in the male relatives of patients with Briquet's syndrome, and led to the suggestion that psychopathy in the male is the phenotypic equivalent of hysteria in the female (Cloninger *et al*, 1975).

In another family study of convicted felons, Cloninger *et al* (1978) found the rate of antisocial personality disorder to be 17% among male relatives of male felons and 4% among female relatives of male felons. Among relatives of female felons, the rate was higher for both men (36%) and women (19%). For both male and female relatives, the rates were substantially higher than in the general population, indicating that the disorder was familial. The authors concluded that the data best-fitted a model of multifactorial transmission. The finding that fewer women in the general population were diagnosed with antisocial personality disorder was explained by gender differences in the threshold for the expression of antisocial behaviour.

Findings from these family studies should be interpreted with caution. Although familial aggregation of a disorder is a necessary prerequisite for the condition to be considered genetic, familiality does not mean that all cases of a disorder must be familial, nor does it imply a genetic basis for inheritance. Better evidence for the heritability of antisocial personality disorder comes from twin and adoption studies.

Twin studies

Until recently, the vast majority of twin studies had only examined criminality. Early studies (e.g. Lange, 1931) appeared to support the role of genetic factors in the transmission of criminality, but variations in ascertainment, zygosity determination and the classification of criminality mean that it is difficult to come to any firm conclusions on the basis of these studies. The introduction of twin registers resulted in greater uniformity in method of ascertainment. In one of the first genetic studies of criminality using a twin register, Christiansen (1974) found that the concordance for criminality was 51% in monozygotic twins compared with 30% in dizygotic twins. Dalgaard & Kringlen (1976) studied 138 twin pairs and found concordance rates of 26% in monozygotic twins and 15% in dizygotic twins. However, after controlling for similarities in environment, they found that monozygotic/dizygotic differences were so reduced that they concluded that "hereditary factors are of no significant importance in the aetiology of common crime".

McGuffin & Gottesman (1984) pooled the results of seven studies of adult criminality and five studies of juvenile delinquency. The weighted-mean concordance for adult criminality in monozygotic twins was 51% and in dizygotic twins was 22%, suggesting a definite genetic contribution. By contrast, for juvenile delinquency there was little difference in the monozygotic:dizygotic concordance rates (87%:72%). It was suggested that while juvenile delinquency is clearly familial, this can be explained primarily by shared environmental influences rather than by genes.

One of the most powerful methods for investigating heritability of a condition is by examining concordance rates for a disorder in monozygotic twins reared apart. Theoretically, resemblance within pairs can be attributed entirely to genetic causes. Grove *et al* (1990) studied 32 sets of monozygotic twins reared apart (median age of separation = 0.2 years). Raters blind to zygosity interviewed the subjects with the DIS in order to determine lifetime diagnoses and symptom counts for antisocial personality disorder and alcohol misuse/dependence. Probandwise diagnostic concordance yielded low estimates for the heritability of these conditions. probably because of the low prevalence of these conditions in the small sample. However, when symptom scores were looked at, both childhood and adult antisocial symptoms showed appreciable between-family variation, and hence significant heritability (heritability of childhood symptoms: 0.4; heritability of adulthood symptoms: 0.28). The significant heritability of childhood antisocial symptoms found in this study is at odds with the findings from McGuffin & Gottesman (1984) and more recent twin data from Thapar & McGuffin (1996), who found that, in a sample of 198 same-sex twin pairs, transmission of antisocial symptoms could be explained entirely by shared environmental factors.

Adoption studies

Theoretically, adoption studies provide the most satisfactory way of examining the respective contributions of environmental and genetic influences in the transmission of a disorder. Adoption studies have been more consistent than twin studies in suggesting a genetic contribution to antisocial behaviour.

Crowe (1972) studied adopted-away children of female felons (a large proportion of whom were assumed to have antisocial personality disorder) and found a significantly greater prevalence of antisocial personality disorder in the offspring of the antisocial personality disorder females compared with control adoptees. Cadoret (1978) reported that adoptees who had antisocial behaviours among relatives were more likely to have antisocial personality disorder. However, other types of psychopathology were also found in these adoptees, supporting the view that antisocial personality disorder belongs to a spectrum of disorders which include somatisation disorder and other cluster B personality disorders (see Lilienfeld *et al*, 1986).

Swedish adoption data have produced mixed findings on the heritability of antisocial behaviour. The initial adoption studies (Bohman, 1978) failed to find evidence for the heritability of criminal behaviour. Subsequent re-analysis (Bohman *et al*, 1982) identified one form of criminality (property offences) that appeared to be inherited. Further analyses of these data (Cloninger *et al*, 1982; Sigvardsson *et al*, 1982) indicate substantial gene–environment interaction in the production of antisocial behaviour; 40% of those from high-risk prenatal backgrounds reared in high-risk homes became petty criminals, as compared with 2.9% of those from neither high-risk biological nor environmental backgrounds. Exposure to an exacerbating environment in the absence of a high-risk biological background was associated with a 6.7% rate of petty criminality, whereas presence of a high-risk biological background without placement in a high-risk environment was associated with a rate of 12.1%.

Danish adoption data have provided a rich source of information for the study of the heritability of antisocial behaviour. Mednick *et al* (1984) examined court convictions in a large sample of Danish adoptees as well as their relatives and found a strong association in convictions for property offences, but not violent crime, between biological parents and adoptive sons. The data showed a positive correlation between numbers of convictions in biological parents and rates of offending in sons. Criminality in the adoptive parents, by contrast, was not associated with criminality in the sons. The Danish adoption data have been re-analysed by several groups. Moffitt (1987) found that 'antisocial disorders' in the biological parents were associated with conviction for property offences in the child. Baker (1986) found high estimates for gene–environment interaction in the production of antisocial behaviour.

A factor that potentially confounds the assessment of the heritability of antisocial behaviour is the presence of alcoholism. Alcohol misuse and dependence have been previously shown to occur frequently in association with antisocial personality disorder. A significant hereditary component has been identified for alcoholism (Goodwin *et al*, 1973) and therefore genetic aetiological factors in antisocial behaviour have to be teased apart from genetic factors related to alcoholism. Many of the earlier genetic studies failed to account for this in their design, and therefore much of the variance in antisocial behaviour could have been explained by the presence of co-occurring alcoholism. In a study of adoptees of antisocial and alcoholic biological relatives, Cadoret *et al* (1985) were able to look specifically at the respective patterns of inheritance for these disorders. In their analysis, antisocial behaviour in first-degree relatives increased the odds of diagnosis of antisocial personality disorder in male adoptees by a factor of 3.7. Among female adoptees, the odds were increased by a factor of 1.9, although the relationship was not statistically significant. A biological background of alcoholism in a first-degree relative increased the odds of diagnosis of alcoholism in male adoptees by a factor of five and in female adoptees by a factor of nine. In contrast, a biological background of alcoholism in a first-degree relative did not increase the risk of antisocial personality disorder among adoptees. The authors concluded that although alcoholism can be regarded as a symptom of antisocial behaviour, with some sociopathic behaviour resulting from alcohol misuse, as far as a common aetiological factor is concerned, it would appear to be genetic with two types of predisposition: one toward alcohol misuse and the other toward antisocial personality.

In conclusion, most twin and adoption studies suggest that antisocial behaviour (crudely defined in terms of criminal convictions) is associated with a moderate degree of heritability. There is also evidence for a substantial degree of genetic–environment interaction in the genesis of antisocial behaviour. There is also evidence for specificity of inheritance of antisocial and alcoholic conditions. The genetic influence appears to be best explained by polygenicity. Given the lack of evidence for single gene effects together with the substantial influence of gene–environment interactions, genetic markers for antisocial behaviour are likely to be of limited discriminatory value. The relevance of these findings to antisocial personality disorder in particular is currently uncertain. In order to answer this question, future genetic studies need to look specifically at samples of operationally-defined personality-disordered subjects.

Childhood antecedents of antisocial personality disorder

A great deal of research indicates that antisocial behaviour in childhood has some continuity with adult antisocial personality disorder and a high continuity with adult social difficulties. Prospective studies of 'deviant' and delinquent children have identified the major risk factors involved in the generation of antisocial and delinquent behaviour. The main findings from some of the more significant studies will be presented.

Prospective studies of 'deviant' children

Childhood conduct disorder

Conduct disorders of childhood are very common (Rutter *et al*, 1975), affecting between 4 and 10% of the population of middle childhood and constituting a third to a half of all referrals to child and adolescent clinics (Robins, 1991). Undoubtedly, the most important longitudinal study of this group is that by Robins (1966). (A summary of Robins' main findings can be found in Chapter 3.) More recent follow-up studies have largely confirmed Robins' findings. Zoccolillo *et al* (1992) examined the effect of conduct disorder on adult social functioning at 26-year follow-up in a sample of 171 young adults who had spent time in care. At follow-up, 40% of conduct-disordered males met DSM–III criteria for antisocial personality disorder, compared with only 43% of those without conduct disorder. In the female group, 35% of those with conduct disorder were diagnosed with antisocial personality disorder compared with none of those without conduct disorder. However, it was apparent that antisocial personality disorder was not the only type of personality disorder that occurred, and that there were continuities to poor social functioning which did not meet criteria for personality disorder. Overall, personality disorder accounted for only about half of the cases of pervasive and persistent social dysfunction in early adult life. The authors concluded that the traditional emphasis on the continuity between conduct disorder and antisocial personality disorder has had unfortunate consequences. The most important consequence has been the underestimation of the relatively poor social outcome in early adult life for children with clinically significant conduct disturbance. The authors went on to argue that the diagnosis of antisocial personality disorder does not provide adequate coverage of the range of disabilities in adult life that are the sequelae of conduct disorder in childhood. This inadequacy, coupled with evidence that conduct symptoms have been reported as antecedents of borderline personality disorder as well as antisocial personality disorder (Soloff & Millward, 1983), led the authors to question the validity of the subcategories of personality disorder.

Storm-Mathisen & Vaglum (1994) have shown the importance of conduct disorder as an antecedent not only for antisocial personality disorder but also for a number of other conditions. Seventy-five consecutive patients with conduct disorder (median age=15 years) were identified from case notes, traced at 19 years, and interviewed with a clinical interview using DSM–III criteria. At follow-up, 33% fulfilled criteria for antisocial personality disorder (*n*=26). In addition, 19 had a substance misuse disorder and 18 a generalised anxiety disorder. On various measures of social functioning, of the 26 people with antisocial personality disorder, 11 had 'fairly good' and 15 'poor' adaptive functioning. The presence of an additional anxiety disorder at entry into the study was a strong predictor of poor outcome.

Childhood hyperactivity

There is a large body of research that has attempted to link childhood hyperactivity with adult antisocial behaviour and, specifically, antisocial personality disorder. (For a detailed review of this area, the reader is referred to Lynam, 1996.) These attempts have, however, been hampered by several methodological problems, including diagnostic heterogeneity at both child and adult levels, and failure to account for the overlap between conduct disorder and hyperactivity (Lilienfeld & Waldman, 1990). The evidence supporting the link comes from two avenues of research – longitudinal studies and genetic studies.

Prospective cohort studies have shown that people diagnosed as hyperactive in childhood show high rates of antisocial behaviour in adolescence and are at high risk of receiving a diagnosis of antisocial personality disorder in adulthood (e.g. Gittelman *et al*, 1985; Weiss & Hechtman, 1986; Mannuzza *et al*, 1993). Retrospective studies (e.g. Morrison, 1980) have supported these results. Unfortunately, the strength of this finding is undermined by the failure of most studies to consider the hypothesis that the association between hyperactivity and antisocial personality disorder is due to the confounding effect of conduct problems. The only way to test this hypothesis effectively is to examine the differential outcomes of groups of children with pure hyperactivity, pure conduct disorder, mixed symptoms of hyperactivity and conduct disorder, and no disorder. Studies that have adopted this approach suggest that the mixed group has the worse outcome, in terms of antisocial behaviour.

Loeber *et al* (1990) looked at these four groups in a sample of 210 boys recruited at 4th, 7th and 10th grades. The boys were followed up after five years and police records were collected. On measures of antisocial behaviour, boys with mixed hyperactivity/conduct problems had the worse outcome, those with conduct problems only were next, those with hyperactivity only next, and finally the remainder of the group. Boys with mixed problems had more police contacts, a higher percentage of multiple offences, a higher rate of offending, and higher self-reported delinquency, aggression and theft.

Farrington *et al* (1990) examined 411 25-year-old men who had been studied extensively since childhood as part of the Cambridge Study of Delinquent Involvement (West & Farrington, 1973, 1977). Using information gathered at 8 and 10 years of age, the investigators established four groups: mixed hyperactive/conduct problems (*n*=59), hyperactivity only (*n*=34), conduct problems only (*n*=40), and comparison (*n*=278). Psychologists, teachers, parents, peers and the boys themselves were used as rating sources. The worst offenders came from the mixed group; for juvenile and adult convictions, the percentages within each group were as follows: 46% and 32% (mixed), 35% and 25% (conduct problems), 24% and 8% (hyperactivity) and 13% and 14% (comparison).

Genetic studies of the association between hyperactivity and antisocial personality disorder have encountered the same methodological problem as that troubling longitudinal studies, that is, the failure to control for the confounding effects of conduct disorder. More recent research has attempted to remedy this problem by comparing the morbid risk of antisocial behaviour in families of conduct-disordered and hyperactive children (e.g. Stewart *et al*, 1980). These studies show that parents of children with hyperactivity are no more likely to receive a diagnosis of antisocial personality disorder than the parents of children without hyperactivity. However, in contrast, the fathers of children with a conduct disorder are more likely to receive a diagnosis of antisocial personality disorder. Studies that have included a mixed sample of hyperactive/conduct-disordered children have found that the risk for antisocial personality disorder is highest among relatives of children in this group (e.g. Lahey *et al*, 1987; Faraone *et al*, 1991).

Finally, in terms of the natural history of antisocial behaviour in samples of hyperactive and conduct-disordered children, many studies have found that, relative to conduct-disordered children, children with mixed disorders have an earlier onset of antisocial behaviour, more frequent, severe and serious antisocial behaviour, and exhibit problems across more settings (e.g. Walker *et al*, 1987; Loeber *et al*, 1990; Moffitt, 1990).

Overall, the evidence suggests that children with disorders characterised by mixed conduct-disorder/hyperactivity symptoms are more likely to receive antisocial personality disorder diagnoses in adulthood, have more antisocial relatives and manifest more frequent, severe and varied patterns of antisocial behaviour, as well as an earlier onset of antisocial behaviour, when compared with their purely hyperactive, purely conduct-disordered and normal counterparts. Lynam (1996) has used the phrase "fledgling psychopath" to describe this group: a group which he believes contains the most likely candidates for future psychopathy.

Studies of the development of delinquency

As noted in the review of natural history studies, knowledge about the natural history of antisocial personality disorder and psychopathy (albeit unsatisfactorily defined in terms of criminal behaviour) has largely been derived from research into crime. In a similar vein, much of our understanding of the risk factors associated with antisocial personality disorder is derived from studies of the development of offending behaviour.

In a series of studies of the development of delinquency, West & Farrington systematically surveyed 411 boys, aged eight years, recruited from a working-class area in London. The results of this survey are extensively documented (West, 1969, 1982; West & Farrington, 1973, 1977; Farrington & West, 1990). The survey is unique in its low attrition rate (94% of those subjects still alive provided information at age 32), use of multiple sources of information, and gathering of information about a wide variety of theoretical constructs.

Briefly, the survey involved repeated interviews and testing at multiple follow-ups between the ages of 8 and 32 years. In addition, repeated searches were carried out in the Central Criminal Record Office in order to provide a comprehensive picture of offending history (excluding minor offences). West & Farrington (1977) developed a series of scales to measure 'antisocial personality' at different ages. Variables were only included in the scales if they were felt to reflect an underlying construct of antisocial personality.

The antisocial personality scales at four ages (10, 14, 18 and 32 years) were all significantly intercorrelated, thus providing evidence for the continuity in antisocial personality from childhood to adulthood. However, what proportion of antisocial children became antisocial adults depended on what cut-off points were used. When the antisocial males were defined as the worst quarter of the sample at each age, it was generally true that about half of those who were antisocial at one age were still antisocial at a later age, and conversely, that about half of those who were antisocial at one age had been antisocial at an earlier age. With more extreme cut-off points, these proportions decreased to about a third or a quarter.

Turning to risk factors for antisocial personality, at age 10 years the strongest correlates of antisocial personality were poor parental supervision, low family income, a delinquent older sibling, low junior school attainment, poor parental child-rearing behaviour (a combination of harsh or erratic discipline, cruel or neglecting attitude and parental disharmony), a lack of interest in the child by the father, large family size, being relatively small in height and transferring to a high delinquency rate secondary school at 11.

Regression analysis was used to establish which risk factors were independent predictors of antisocial personality. At age 10, the independently important risk factors were poor parental supervision, low junior school attainment, poor parental child-rearing behaviour and high neuroticism. At 14 years, in addition to antisocial personality at age 10, the independently important predictors of antisocial personality were separation from a parent, low non-verbal IQ, not having many friends and low junior school attainment. At 18, in addition to antisocial personality at 14, the independently important predictors of antisocial personality were having a convicted parent at age 10, the father not involved in the boy's leisure activities at age 12, periodic unemployment of the father at age 14, the father not staying on at school beyond the minimum school-leaving age, the boy not staying on at school beyond the minimum school-leaving age, and not having many friends. In the assessment of risk factors, an attempt was made to distinguish between 'indicators' of antisocial personality and risk factors, although, as Farrington acknowledges, it is not unambiguously clear in all cases that the risk factors are possible causes of antisocial personality, as opposed to consequences or indicators.

The survey also revealed the protective influence of having few friends. Farrington *et al* (1988) investigated the vulnerable boys who were not convicted up to age 32, and found that the most character-istic feature of these boys was that they had few or no friends at age eight. At 32, while they were 'well-behaved', they were often leading relatively unsuccessful lives.

Farrington (1990) concluded that the most important independent predictors of convictions fell into six categories: socio-economic depri-vation, poor child-rearing, antisocial family members, school failure, impulsivity and antisocial child behaviour. All of the significant risk factors fell into one of these categories. On the basis of the results of the Cambridge Survey, Farrington (1986, 1992, 1993) has proposed a theory to explain the development of offending, and which might be used to explain the development of antisocial behaviour.

Studies of childhood temperament

Temperament is an important determinant of behavioural continuity over time, and is therefore highly relevant to a discussion of the development of antisocial personality. The term temperament is generally defined as personality traits with at least some continuity over time, which appear in early childhood and have a constitutional, largely genetic basis (Plomin *et al*, 1988). The New York Longitudinal Study (Chess & Thomas, 1984) explored temperament with detailed interview and observational methods from infancy to adult life. Nine dimensions of temperament were identified, of which four were relatively stable over time. Other work based on factor analyses of parental questionnaires has suggested that four aspects of normal temperament are largely genetically determined: emotionality, activity level, sociability and impulsivity (Buss & Plomin, 1975). High levels of the last three of these four elements significantly contribute to the development of aggressive and antisocial behaviour. (More recently, Caspi & Silva (1995) have refined the classification of childhood temperament into three types: 'undercontrolled', 'inhibited' and 'well-adjusted'.)

A large literature has established that aggression is one of the most stable forms of behaviour over time, particularly in boys. Olweus (1979) reviewed 16 studies of aggression with time-lags ranging from 6 months to 21 years. The disattenuated stability coefficients ranged from 0.98 for Olweus' (1977) own study of 85 13-year-olds in Sweden over one year, to 0.36 for Kagan & Moss' (1962) study of 36 five-year-olds. Olweus (1978) found that stability coefficients generally decreased linearly with lag and that stabilities were greater for older boys than younger boys.

Roff & Wirt (1984) followed a sample of over 1000 low peer-status boys and girls through archival record sources into young adulthood. The authors found that primary school measures of aggression were significantly related to later delinquency and criminal behaviour for males but not for females. In a 20-year follow-up study of Swedish children aged 10, 13 and 15 years, Magnusson (1988) attempted to trace antecedents of adult criminality. Specific variables were examined: hyperactive and aggressive childhood behaviours, and low adrenaline excretion at 13 years. All three were significantly related to adult criminality, and almost half the boys rated as extremely aggressive at 13 had recorded crimes at 18–26 years.

Huesmann *et al* (1984) have produced evidence for not only stability of aggression in individuals across time, but also for stability of aggression across generations. Six hundred subjects were recruited at eight years of age and childhood aggression was rated using a peer-nominated index of aggression. Parent aggression was derived from the parent rating of severity of punishment used in response to misdeeds by the subject. At 22-year follow-up, indications of the subject's aggression were derived from self-ratings, spouse ratings, and criminal justice scores of the total number of convictions in the previous 10 years. The 22-year stability coefficients for aggression within individuals were 0.5 for boys and 0.34 for girls. Aggression and IQ at age eight were moderately correlated negatively (–0.27 for boys and –0.32 for girls). Aggressiveness predicted serious antisocial behaviour (including criminality), spouse abuse and self-reported physical aggression in adult life. The stability of aggression at comparable ages across generations in the same family (measured in terms of parental punitiveness and aggressiveness of subjects and their children) was even more stable than within individuals.

In summary, therefore, there is substantial evidence for the continuity of dimensions of temperament over time. In particular, aggression (which is partially determined by temperament) displays stability across time within individuals and also across generations. Recently, evidence has emerged that specifically tests a link between temperamental 'deviance' in childhood and adult psychiatric disorder, and specifically antisocial personality disorder. As part of the Dunedin Multidisciplinary Health and Development Study, Caspi *et al* (1996) classified a sample of 1037 three-year-old children into one of five temperamental groups: 'undercontrolled' (irritable and impulsive), 'inhibited' (socially reticent), 'well-adjusted' (within normal limits for age), 'confident' (eager to explore) and 'reserved' (timid and uncomfortable in the testing situation). At 21 years, over 90% of the sample (attrition rate 7.3%) were interviewed with the DIS to obtain diagnoses of mental disorder. In addition, an assessment of impairment and an informant index of mental health were obtained, and computerised conviction records were sought. Overall, undercontrolled (46%) and inhibited (53%) children were the most likely to be diagnosed with psychiatric disorder. More specifically, undercontrolled children were 2.9 times more likely to be diagnosed with antisocial personality disorder ($P < 0.05$; 95% CI 1.1–8.1), 2.2 times as likely to be recidivistic offenders ($P < 0.05$; 95% CI 1.1–4.7), and 4.5 times as likely to be convicted for a violent offence ($P < 0.01$; 95% CI 1.8–10.9). These data indicate that in the absence of significant characterological change, early-appearing behavioural differences may act as a persisting risk factor for antisocial personality disorder.

Childhood experiential antecedents of antisocial behaviour

Patients with personality disorders frequently report disturbing and often traumatic childhood experiences. In a study of potential aetiological factors for axis II disorders in patients with antisocial personalities in special hospitals and prisons, Coid (1992) found that the early history of 80% of subjects was characterised by various forms of deprivation. Almost half had witnessed discord between parental figures involving repeated physical violence, 42% had been raised in conditions of material poverty, 42% had experienced physical abuse themselves, 40% had been placed in the care of social services due to family breakdown, and over a third had lost a parent through divorce or death. Nineteen per cent had violent or criminal parents, 24% were sexually abused by family members, and in female psychopaths incest occurred in 28%. Coid's group consisted of extremely disturbed subjects, and hence the generalisability of the findings is limited, although the study does provide some idea of the range of childhood traumata experienced by individuals with severe personality disorder.

A multitude of adverse environmental factors have been shown to interfere with the normal process of child development. These include psychiatric disorder in parents (especially personality disorder), marital discord, loss of parents, large family size, institutional care of the child, inconsistent discipline, criminality in parents, and a chaotic family environment. Naturally, many of these factors act non-specifically in the pathogenesis of a variety of axis I and axis II disorders, and, in addition, are risk factors for the development of juvenile delinquency and adult criminality. Many adverse risk factors are so confounded by their association with other consequential adversities that any specific contribution to a disorder is not readily traced. The aetiology of antisocial personality disorder is likely to involve complex interactional effects between a variety of factors within the developing child, the parents, and the social environment, operating within a multivariate causal framework. In addition to the problems posed by this complex theoretical framework, much of the literature on specific associations between early adversity and axis II categories has been based on weak methodology characterised by unsystematic observation, overdependence on self-report and retrospective data, a reliance on highly disturbed samples of subjects, and infrequent use of baseline data from control groups. More recently, however, studies employing improved methodology have clarified the relationship between some early experiential factors and antisocial behaviour.

Childhood victimisation

The impact of abuse/neglect on the victim has been the focus of numerous studies with varying degrees of methodological rigour. A wide range of consequences of childhood victimisation has been demonstrated, such as conduct disorder (Friedrich & Luecke, 1988), substance misuse (Herman, 1986), aggressiveness (Zeiller, 1982), antisocial behaviour (Oliver, 1988), delinquency, criminality and violent behaviour (Widom, 1989).

One of the most pervasive claims in academic and popular writings of the 1970s and 1980s referred to the so-called 'cycle of violence' (i.e. that abused children become abusers and victims of violence become violent offenders). Much of the empirical evidence underlying this claim was contradictory and reliant on weak methodology. Widom (1989) provided one of the first rigorous tests of the cycle of violence hypothesis, using operationalised definitions of abuse, a prospective design and a control group. Nine hundred and eight children aged 11 years or under who had been abused/neglected were recruited from cases of abuse/neglect processed and substantiated by a juvenile court. These children were compared with a non-victimised group of children matched for age, gender, race and place of residence, and followed prospectively into young adulthood (average age at follow-up 26 years). At follow-up, in comparison with controls, abused/neglected children had more arrests as a juvenile (26 v. 17%), more arrests as an adult (29 v. 21%) and more arrests for any violent offence (11 v. 8%). After logistic regression analysis, however, although childhood victimisation remained a predictor of violent criminal behaviour, it was not as powerful a predictor as the socio-demographic characteristics of gender, age and race.

Luntz & Widom (1994) have looked more specifically at the extent to which having been abused/neglected in childhood raises a person's risk for having antisocial personality disorder. Four hundred and sixteen abused/neglected children from Widom's original cohort were matched with a group of 283 non-victimised children and followed prospectively into adulthood (average age at follow-up 27.5 years). Subjects were interviewed with the DIS in order to determine the lifetime prevalence of antisocial personality disorder in the two groups. At follow-up, significantly more of the abused/neglected male subjects met criteria for antisocial personality disorder (13.5 v. 7.1%); the difference for women was non-significant. The difference for men remained significant even when gender, age, socio-economic status and criminal history were controlled for.

Clearly an important factor which may confound the association between early victimisation and adult antisocial behaviour is paternal alcoholism. Few studies have looked at the interactive combinations of paternal alcoholism and child abuse on antisocial behaviour. Pollock *et al* (1990) attempted to address this issue in a survey of sons of fathers with alcoholism; 131 subjects from a Danish perinatal birth cohort, whose fathers had received hospital treatment for alcoholism, were interviewed with a detailed structured interview in order to obtain information on life crises including repeated physical attacks. Antisocial behaviour was determined systematically by clinical interview, and the Danish National Police Register was screened for crimes. Logistic regression analysis showed that more sons of fathers with alcoholism than comparison subjects reported that they had been physically beaten, although this difference was non-significant. When paternal alcoholism was controlled for, self-reported history of being beaten by a parent as a child was predictive of five out of the six antisocial variables. Although the data rely heavily on self-report, they suggest that paternal alcoholism and childhood victimisation may represent independent phenomena.

Coercive child-rearing

There is evidence that harsh or rejecting parenting is linked to conduct disorder (Wolkind & Rutter, 1985), and also that the level of monitoring and supervision by parents plays a significant role in the development of antisocial behaviour (Crowell, 1993). Faulty parenting technique can be passed from one generation to another (Olweus, 1979), thus perpetuating the transmission of aggression across generations. Patterson (1982) has attempted to explain the development of childhood aggression in terms of a mutually reinforcing coercive process between parents and child. It is proposed that children with a difficult temperament are at greatest risk of evoking such coercive responses, whereas parents most at risk of responding coercively are the socio-economically deprived, especially when depressed, under stress, or under the influence of drugs.

A neglected area of study has been the identification of potential protective factors. These may be defined as dispositional attributes, environmental conditions, or positive events that mitigate against early negative experience (Garmezy, 1981). In the Cambridge Delinquency Survey, forming a stable relationship with a wife or girlfriend and moving away from inner London (a high crime area) both made the continuation of a delinquent career less likely. The Kauai longitudinal study (Werner & Smith, 1982) has provided valuable information on factors that either promote or mitigate against an adverse adult outcome. Factors within the environment included the presence of key 'other persons' such as close peers and teachers, and additional caregivers besides the mother.

6 Social and health care burden of antisocial personality disorder

The reviewed literature has shown that antisocial personality disorder is a severe persistent disorder commonly found in criminal populations and one which often occurs in association with other psychiatric conditions, particularly disorders of addiction. The limited data on natural history suggest that it is a disorder with a poor prognosis, characterised by a multitude of social problems. This chapter examines the nature of the burden associated with antisocial personality disorder.

Before tackling this subject, an important problem with the definition of personality disorder needs first to be considered. Social and personal disruption are defining features of all personality disorders. However, this definition fails to distinguish between symptoms (i.e. impairment) and the psychosocial consequences of those symptoms (i.e. handicap). The consequence of this is a rather circular position whereby the disorder is defined in terms of handicap – handicap which is itself the result of the disorder being defined. The problem is not unique to the personality disorders, and represents an inherent weakness of psychiatric classification (McFarlane, 1988). One solution to this problem would be to adopt a definition of personality disorder that limits itself to impairment (i.e. personality traits), and to consider associated disability and handicap quite separately. This sort of approach is advocated by the International Classification of Impairments, Disabilities and Handicaps (World Health Organization, 1980) although perhaps, disappointingly, it is one which has as yet failed to have a significant impact on clinical practice. Antisocial personality disorder exemplifies the circularity inherent in current definitions of personality disorder, as, in addition to the necessary 'burden criterion', the whole definition emphasises antisocial behaviour. Therefore studies that try to examine the nature of this burden, in terms of indices such as unemployment, crime and service usage, usually come to the rather unilluminating conclusion that antisocial personality disorder is associated with a heavy burden.

85

The study of the burden of antisocial personality disorder is effectively the study of the natural history of the disorder, a subject of which we know embarrassingly little. In its place, a great deal of literature exists dedicated to the minutiae of burden, for example, studies of the diagnostic profile of the homeless or unemployed. Such studies do not provide a representative picture of the burden of a disorder – they merely indicate its prevalence in a range of diverse populations. Furthermore, very few studies have attempted to examine a range of social disturbance associated with a range of disorders. One exception is Thompson & Bland's (1995) survey of mental disorder and associated social dysfunction in a Canadian household population. As part of the Edmonton Community Survey (Bland *et al*, 1988*a*), 3258 randomly selected household residents were interviewed with the DIS in order to establish prevalence rates of mental disorder and associated social disturbance. Eight social problems were selected for study, and in order to safeguard against the possibility of spurious associations, antisocial personality disorder was only determined in the absence of the defining statements for all social problems, except suicide attempts. Each social problem showed a significant relationship with the majority of individual disorders, although of note is the fact that the odds of exhibiting antisocial personality disorder for each of the social problems was greater than for any of the other disorders. The odds ratios associated with antisocial personality disorder for each problem were: alcohol misuse, 37; drug misuse, 17.5; divorce, 7.8; unemployment, 5.9; suicide attempt, 17.6; felony, 22.6; spouse abuse, 8.3; and child abuse, 9.5 (for all the odds ratios quoted, $P < 0.001$).

Studies of selected populations indicate that antisocial personality disorder is especially prevalent among the unemployed, homeless, wife batterers and child abusers. The findings of studies of these selected groups are summarised in Table 6.1.

An important facet of social burden is crime, although the accurate assessment of this form of burden is conflated by current operationalised definitions of psychopathy which emphasise antisocial behaviour. Two studies have focused on antisocial personality disorder and demonstrated a high degree of association with crime and, in particular, violent crime. Hodgins *et al* (1996) used Danish registries to identify a birth cohort and to document all psychiatric admissions and all criminal proceedings of the 324 401 members of this cohort up to age 43 years. Persons who had been admitted to a psychiatric ward were assigned to a diagnostic category according to a hierarchy of principal discharge diagnoses. They were then compared with other persons never admitted to a psychiatric ward with regard to the prevalence, type and frequency of criminal convictions. For both men and women,

TABLE 6.1
Studies of the burden of antisocial personality disorder

Study	Sample	Measures	Findings
Bland & Orn (1986)	1200 randomly selected adult household residents	DIS	2.6% admitted to abusing a child. 49% of those who were violent had antisocial personality disorder, recurrent depression and/or alcoholism. Antisocial personality disorder + alcohol: 48 times more likely to commit family violence
Bland *et al* (1988*b*)	3258 randomly selected adult household residents	DIS	Lifetime prevalence of all psychiatric disorders higher in unemployed group. Odds ratio of unemployment given antisocial personality disorder 6.2
Koegel *et al* (1988)	379 homeless adults	DIS	Lifetime prevalence of antisocial personality disorder 21%. Antisocial personality disorder 4 times more likely in homeless population
Dinwiddie & Bucholz (1993)	1869 St Louis ECA sample	DIS	4% admitted to child abuse. Abusers more likely to receive diagnosis of antisocial personality disorder, alcohol misuse or depression
Dinwiddie (1992)	(a) 61 wife batterers (b) 319 controls	HELPER	Prevalence of antisocial personality disorder (Feighner criteria): (a) 46%; (b) 31% Odds ratio: 1.9 (95% CI 1.0–3.6)
Else *et al* (1993)	21 wife batterers, 21 controls	MMPI	Batterers scored higher than controls on measures of antisocial and borderline personality disorder
Hart *et al* (1993)	85 wife assaulters	MCMI–II PDE	MCMI–II: 90% had a personality disorder; PDE: 29% antisocial personality disorder

DIS, Diagnostic Interview Schedule; HELPER, Home Environment and Lifetime Psychiatric Evaluation Record; MMPI, Minnesota Multiphasic Personality Inventory; MCMI–II, Millon Clinical Multiaxial Inventory–II; PDE, Personality Disorder Examination.

all diagnostic groups were found to be at significantly increased risk for all types of crime compared with the non-disordered group. For the period 1978–1990 (when police data recording was computerised and, therefore, more accurate), the estimated relative risk of committing a crime given a diagnosis of antisocial personality disorder was 6.5 (95% CI 5.9–7.1) for female subjects and 5.3 (95%

CI 5.0–5.6) for male subjects. The estimated relative risk for registering for at least one violent crime was 12.2 (95% CI 8.8–16.9) for female subjects and 7.2 (95% CI 6.5–8.0) for male subjects.

Eronen *et al* (1996) examined the forensic psychiatric records of 693 Finnish homicide offenders, in order to generate DSM–III and DSM–III–R diagnoses. The prevalences of mental disorders were then used to calculate odds ratios for the statistical increase in risk associated with specific mental disorders. The odds ratio of homicidal violence given a diagnosis of antisocial personality disorder was 53.8 (95% CI 28.5–101.5) for women and 11.7 (95% CI 9.5–14.4) for men.

Both studies relied on a retrospective design and took place in settings with relatively homogeneous populations, low overall crime rates, and relatively uniform prosperity – characteristics that are very different from those of the UK. These facts limit the generalisability of the findings, and it would be of interest to see whether a prospective study in the UK would be able to replicate these findings.

As discussed previously, the PCL provides an alternative approach to the conceptualisation of psychopathy, focusing on both person-ality traits central to traditional conceptions of psychopathy, and behavioural manifestations of the chaotic lifestyle. Predictive criterion-related evidence for the validity of the PCL also provides information on the crime-related burden of psychopathy, while overcoming some of the tautologies experienced by studies that have adopted antisocial personality disorder. Using the PCL, Hare & Jutai (1983) have shown that, compared with non-psychopathic criminals, psychopathic criminals are likely to commit a greater amount of crime. In addition, psychopaths are more likely to use violent and aggressive behaviour than are criminals in general (Hare & McPherson, 1984). Compared with the diagnoses of alcohol misuse or schizophrenia, a high psychopathy score is more strongly related to the likelihood of violent recidivism (Rice & Harris, 1995). Finally, among sex offenders, psychopathy scores have been found to be significantly related to recidivism for both violent offences in general and sexual offences in particular (Rice *et al*, 1990). Using the PCL to predict who will commit greater amounts of crime, however, creates tautologies of its own. Table 1 in the Introduction shows that included among the items on the PCL are "criminal versatility" and "revocation of conditional release". It should therefore come as no surprise to find that PCL-positive subjects commit a greater amount of crime and are more aggressive compared with "non-psychopaths".

Studies of health service utilisation patterns indicate that individ-uals with personality disorders are frequent users of health services (Saarento *et al*, 1997), although the literature on antisocial personality disorder in this respect is sparse. In a naturalistic follow-up study of 91 subjects, Perry *et al* (1985) found that subjects with borderline and antisocial personality disorders and bipolar II affective disorders all used psychiatric care frequently, and that individuals with borderline personality disorder used the highest levels of care over time. Leaf *et al* (1985) examined factors related to out-patient use of mental health services, including the probability that a person with a DIS-diagnosed mental disorder would make any use of mental health services in the previous six months, and the number of visits for these services. Having a diagnosis of antisocial personality disorder increased the odds of having a mental health visit in the previous six months by almost six times, although, among those treated, individuals with antisocial personality disorder had relatively few visits to services. ECA data on mental health service usage by people with mental disorders indicate that while persons whose primary complaint is antisocial personality disorder constitute only a small proportion of the total number of mentally disordered persons presenting (3%), the one-year visit rate of these individuals is among the highest, with a rate of 26.4 visits per person (Narrow *et al*, 1993). (Given the high degree of association between antisocial personality disorder and drug-use disorders and the relatively large number of persons presenting for drug-related problems, the actual amount of service usage for persons with antisocial personality disorder is likely to be far higher than that estimated.)

In most countries, including the UK, issues of scarcity and rationing in the health care sector are the perennial subject of debate. These debates have led to an increasing preoccupation with the costs associated with illness and a striving for economic efficiency in resource usage. Quantification of the economic burden sustained from a disorder is now possible using a variety of techniques. These include cost–benefit analysis, cost–utility analysis, cost-effectiveness analysis and cost of illness analysis. Of these, the cost of illness approach is of greatest relevance to the present discussion. Cost of illness studies measure the impact of the burden of disease as quantified by resources used to treat and care for a condition. Most of the cost of illness literature deals with the economic burden of axis I disorders, and in fact no cost of illness studies of antisocial personality disorder were identified by the literature search. Only one cost of illness study has looked at personality disorders in general. Using UK national prevalence data, and data on service usage, Smith *et al* (1995) estimated that in 1986 the NHS spent £61.24 million on personality disorders. This figure is over four times that spent on substance and alcohol misuse. Figures obtained in this way provide only a crude estimate of burden, as they do not account for lost productivity at work, or indeed broader psychosocial costs, such as distress to self and others. Also, the estimates are only as good as the estimates of prevalence of a condition. Another problem associated with the cost of illness approach is that it provides an attempt to estimate resource savings and increased length and quality of life if the condition under consideration was eliminated. It has been argued that as the possibility of the total eradication of a disease is remote, cost of illness studies are of limited policy relevance (Shiell *et al*, 1987). Given the limited understanding of the aetiological and protective factors associated with various personality disorders, this latter point is perhaps especially relevant.

7   Needs assessment

One important role of epidemiology is the analysis of health services in order to aid planning of future service provision (Morris, 1957). In recent years, there has been a shift of emphasis from service-led to needs-led provision (Slade & Thornicroft, 1995). The NHS and Community Care Act 1990 recognises that the long-term mentally ill have multiple needs, and, under this legislation, local authorities now have a statutory obligation to assess the physical, psychological and social needs of these individuals. The assessment of need is, therefore, an important component of service planning and hence also epidemiology.

This chapter summarises the literature on needs assessment, discusses the approaches currently available for assessing needs, and considers the application of these approaches to patients with antisocial personality disorder.

Defining need

There is at present no consensus on how need should be defined (Holloway, 1994). Definitions have been proposed from a variety of disciplines including psychology, sociology, medicine and public health.

Thornicroft *et al* (1996) noted that the *Oxford English Dictionary* offers "necessity, requirement and essential". From the field of psychology, Maslow (1954) described a "hierarchy of needs" which extend from basic physiological needs, through needs for safety, love and self-esteem, to "self-actualisation" needs. Bradshaw (1972) produced a taxonomy of social need which distinguishes four separate definitions of need as used by service managers and researchers. These were 'normative need' (i.e. what experts define as need), 'felt' need (the wants and desires of service users), expressed need (the demand for service) and 'comparative' need (the gap in service provision between one area and another, with weighting for differences in local morbidity). Matthew (1971) differentiated between medical 'need', 'demand' and 'utilisation'. According to Matthew, a need for medical care exists "when an individual has an illness or disability for which there is effective and acceptable treatment or care". Finally, from the public health perspective, Stevens & Gabbay (1991) distinguished between 'need' (what people benefit from), 'demand' (what people ask for) and 'supply' (what is provided). Different disciplines, therefore, may use the word 'need' to mean quite different things. Inevitably, such confusion over the meaning of the term can cause a psychiatric team considerable problems in establishing a cogent philosophy for the delivery of care. Holloway (1994) described two models of need in community care (implicit and psychiatric), and proposed that differences between these models can reduce communication between psychiatrists and community staff.

Measurement of need

Two levels of needs assessment can be distinguished: the population and the individual.

Population-based assessments

Population-based assessments inform the development, planning and evaluation of services (Slade & Thornicroft, 1995). Ideally, the best way to establish the actual needs of a population is to undertake an epidemiological survey. However, few epidemiological studies have incorporated an assessment of the population's needs. Some of the recent prison surveys have incorporated assessments of the unmet treatment of sentenced and remand prisoners. For example, Maden *et al* (1994) estimated that 6% of the remand population would require long-term treatment for personality disorder, and that about half of all remand inmates with a primary diagnosis of personality disorder would benefit from further treatment and assessment for a therapeutic community. Few epidemiological studies have, however, adopted this sort of approach, and since comprehensive epidemiological data on need are lacking at the population level, proxy measures such as prevalence data and service use or social deprivation indicators are often used instead.

Epidemiological surveys can be useful in estimating the likely burden of a disorder in a population, and thus provide indirect evidence of needs for treatment; indeed, this was a major purpose of the ECA studies. Bebbington (1992) argued, however, that establishing prevalence can only be regarded as a first step in the assessment of the needs for treatment in the general population. The major limitation of this approach is that it assumes that subjects in the community need treatment merely because they meet symptomatic case criteria. Bebbington argued that instruments measuring caseness do not adequately assess impairment in social performance, which should be measured separately. Similarly, studies of health service use provide only crude estimates of the population's need for treatment. First, the data on which service figures are based are generally unreliable. Second, not all of those in need will use services (Goldberg & Huxley, 1980) and, moreover, not all of those who use services are in need of them. In the light of the deficiencies of current epidemiological data, it has been argued that there is a need for a "fourth generation" of epidemiological surveys with a direct focus on the evaluation of the need for specific treatments and the services within which they are most appropriately provided (Bebbington *et al*, 1996).

Individual assessments of need

Over recent years, a considerable number of needs assessment schedules have been developed, although the issue of how best to make an individual assessment of need remains unresolved. Early attempts focused on the assessment of symptoms, although, as noted previously, this approach lacks validity in predicting requirements for services. More recently, attempts have been made to assess disability and social performance (Wykes & Sturt, 1986), needs for services (Clifford *et al*, 1991) and needs for action by mental health teams (Brewin *et al*, 1987; Phelan *et al*, 1995). Three main schedules will be discussed in detail: the MRC Needs for Care Assessment, the Cardinal Needs Schedule and the Camberwell Assessment of Needs.

MRC Needs for Care Assessment

The MRC Needs for Care Assessment schedule (Brewin *et al*, 1987) was developed specifically for measuring the needs of the long-term mentally ill living in the community and in touch with psychiatric services. It is based on the following definition of need for care. A need is present when:

(a) functioning falls below or threatens to fall below some minimum specified level; and
(b) this is due to a remediable or potentially remediable cause.

The schedule involves two distinct stages of data collection, which are summarised in Fig. 7.1. In the first stage, 20 areas of clinical and social functioning are assessed using a number of standardised instruments. (Clinical areas of functioning include items such as the presence of symptoms and side-effects of medication. Social areas of functioning include items such as personal cleanliness, shopping and cooking skills.) In the second stage, a member of staff is questioned about a standard list of items of care relevant to each identified problem. Questioning includes details of whether each item of care has been tried, and about its appropriateness, effectiveness and acceptability to the patient. Judgements of the primary need status follow algorithmically from these ratings.

Under this scheme:

(a) a need is *met* when it has attracted some at least partially effective items of care, and when no other items of care of greater potential effectiveness exist;

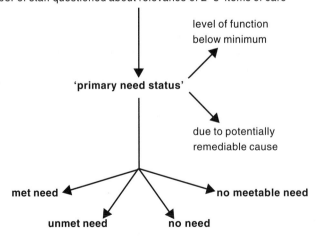

1. Assessment of 20 areas of clinical and social functioning – using standardised instruments (Present State Examination, Social Behaviour Scale, Mini-Mental State Examination, Abnormal Involuntary Movements Scale, education and medical questionnaire)

↓

'problem'

2. Member of staff questioned about relevance of 2–8 'items of care'

level of function
below minimum

'primary need status'

due to potentially
remediable cause

met need ← | → no meetable need

unmet need   no need

Fig. 7.1   MRC Needs for Care Assessment

(b) a need is *unmet* when it has attracted only a partly effective or no item of care, and when other items of care of greater potential effectiveness exist;

(c) a need is *unmeetable* when no effective items of care are currently available.

A considerable number of studies have now used this schedule, and its psychometric properties are reported to be excellent (Brewin & Wing, 1993), although estimates of validity are limited given that no other comparable definitions and measures of need exist. The schedule does, however, have its critics. Hogg & Marshall (1992) found the schedule to be excessively time-consuming (it can take between 3–5 hours to complete), and have argued that it fails to account fully for the views of staff and relatives. The Cardinal Needs Schedule was developed specifically to tackle these perceived shortcomings.

Cardinal Needs Schedule

This is a modification of the MRC Needs for Care approach. It is shorter, easier to use, and purports to take systematic account of the views of patients and their carers (Marshall *et al*, 1995). Using a similar algorithm to the one displayed in Fig. 7.1, it identifies 'cardinal problems' as those that satisfy three criteria:

(1) the 'cooperation criterion' (the patient is willing to accept help for the problem);

(2) the 'carer stress criterion' (the problem causes considerable stress or inconvenience to people caring for the patient);

(3) the 'severity criterion' (the problem endangers the health or safety of the patient, or the safety of others).

To rate this schedule, data are collected using the Manchester Scale for mental state assessment (Krawiecka *et al*, 1977), the REHAB scale (Baker & Hall, 1988), and a specially developed additional information questionnaire (Marshall *et al*, 1995). Patients' views are rated using the Client Opinion Interview and the Carer Stress Interview (Marshall *et al*, 1995). A computerised version has also been developed.

Camberwell Assessment of Need (CAN)

This is a clinically-orientated instrument (Phelan *et al*, 1995), designed specifically to assist local authorities in their fulfilment of statutory obligations under the NHS and Community Care Act 1990. It aims to provide a comprehensive assessment of a wide range of human needs by incorporating the views of both patient and staff.

Because it is comparatively quick and straightforward to use, it is suitable for use by a wide range of clinical staff and therefore, in theory, can be incorporated into routine clinical practice. Two main versions of the instrument are currently available: a clinical version designed primarily for use by staff to plan patients' care, and a research version designed primarily as a mental health service evaluation tool. In addition, the authors are currently piloting a shorter version – the Camberwell Assessment of Need Short Appraisal Schedule (CANSAS). The psychometric properties of the CAN have now been established (Phelan *et al*, 1995) and been found to be satisfactory. The instrument is being translated into several other languages, and is being published in a computer version.

Assessment of the needs of mentally disordered offenders and psychopaths

The assessment of need has become an increasingly prominent issue in the development of services for mentally disordered offenders. In 1991, the Government recommended that regional health authorities should ensure a regular assessment of the needs of their residents for secure provision, and of the non-secure hospital needs of their mentally disordered offenders. The Special Hospitals Service Authority issued service guidelines for patients with personality disorder that include "an assessment of needs in the National Health Service and Criminal Justice System" (Special Hospitals Service Authority, 1995). Finally, the Reed Report (Department of Health & Home Office, 1994) emphasised the need to care for mentally disordered offenders, and as a result central capital allocation for medium-secure developments was increased.

In spite of a mounting preoccupation with the needs of mentally disordered offenders, very few systematic approaches have been developed to allow the systematic assessment of the unique needs of this specific group. The PRiSM team, in conjunction with the Department of Forensic Psychiatry, at the Institute of Psychiatry have recently developed a Forensic Version of the Camberwell Assessment of Need (CAN–F; Bindman, personal communication, 1998) and are currently piloting the instrument. The areas of potential need included in the CAN–F are listed in Table 7.1. The CAN–F bears a close resemblance to the original instrument and the approach is identical. There are, however, questions relating to specific offences, and for some areas of potential need the subject is specifically asked to make a judgement as to how much, in their view, problems in a particular area contributed to the index offence or incident leading to the current admission. Security needs are also explicitly dealt with

TABLE 7.1
*Areas of potential need included in the CAN–F (Camberwell
Assessment of Need – Forensic Version). (CAN: Phelan et al,1995;
forensic adaptation: Bindman, personal communication, 1998)*

Accommodation
Food
Looking after the living environment
Self-care
Daytime activities
Physical health
Psychotic symptoms
Information about condition and treatment
Psychological distress
Safety to self
Safety to others
Alcohol
Drugs
Company
Intimate relationships
Sexual expression
Childcare
Basic education
Telephone
Transport
Money
Benefits
Insight
Sexual offences
Arson

by the CAN–F under the problem categories 'safety to self' and 'safety to others'.

Recent collaborative work between the forensic adolescent team at Prestwich Hospital, Manchester, and the University of Manchester has led to the development of a needs assessment schedule for adolescents (further details available from the author upon request). The aim of the schedule is to assess the social and psychiatric needs of young people (13–18 years) with chronic challenging behaviours such as aggression and offending. It follows a very similar approach to the one employed by the Cardinal Needs Schedule. The first step is the quantification of four functional areas:

(a) severity of 21 problem areas;
(b) the young person's motivation for help with their problems;
(c) the levels of stress of carers resulting from each of the problem areas;
(d) the help offered to deal with these problems and its acceptability and effectiveness.

Consideration of (a), (b) and (c) results in a decision being made as to whether a cardinal problem exists. This cardinal problem is then matched against help offered (d), using a panel of clinicians. If the help offered does not address the cardinal problem, then a cardinal need is said to exist and options are given as to how best to offer help for this cardinal need. The schedule's discriminant validity is in the process of being determined by testing on three groups: youths attending court, those in secure units and a psychiatric out-patient group. Although primarily intended as a needs assessment schedule for young people, the team are considering adapting it for adult forensic samples.

The recent prison surveys presented in the review have highlighted the high rates of psychiatric morbidity in prisoners and have found that large numbers of both remand and sentenced prisoners have treatment needs (Gunn *et al*, 1991; Maden *et al*, 1994). Large numbers of personality-disordered prisoners were found to have unmet treatment needs, with many judged to require assessment for a therapeutic community. These needs, however, deserve closer scrutinisation. Brewin (1992) has categorised needs into: needs for health, needs for services and needs for action/care. The first category equates need with social disablement and impaired functioning. The second category assumes that some needs require services. The third category is based on the assumption that needs are alleviated by intervention. Personality disorders are usually accompanied by multiple social, psychological and medical problems. The review has shown that, for individuals with antisocial personality disorder, these include substance misuse and homelessness – problems for which there are effective interventions. Using the sort of problem-seeking approach adopted by needs assessment instruments such as the CAN, a list of further problems with potentially remediable causes can be established for individuals with antisocial personality disorder and other personality disorders. These would, therefore, be problems that equate with needs for health, services and action under Brewin's scheme. On the other hand, while it is clear that individuals with personality disorder and specifically antisocial personality disorder have a need for health (i.e. they are a disabled group with a reduced level of functioning), it currently remains unclear as to whether their core psychological disturbance is amenable to treatment. In their recent review of the treatment of psychopathy and antisocial personality disorder, Dolan & Coid (1993) concluded that: " ... there is still no convincing evidence that psychopaths can or cannot be treated". There are, of course, humanitarian considerations imposing a sense of moral obligation on doctors to provide care for a group of individuals who are clearly psychologically disturbed. However, until the vexed issue of treatability is resolved, their treatment needs remain unclear. At present, therefore, it would seem that in the language of the MRC Needs for Care Assessment schedule, the defining psychological disturbance of personality disorder would equate with the category of 'no meetable need'.

8   Conclusions and recommendations

As was noted in the Introduction, the literature on antisocial and dissocial personality disorder has been considered together with that on the older diagnostic equivalents of these terms – psychopathy and sociopathy. This was done to maximise the yield of literature and is entirely consistent with the view that antisocial personality disorder represents an attempt to operationalise the concept of psychopathy. (Whether indeed psychopathy is a concept worthy of operationalising remains the subject of continuing debate.) By collating this literature, an epidemiological picture for antisocial personality disorder has been built-up. The picture is one of a disorder which is relatively common in community samples, more common in criminals, and one which has major public health implications in terms of its association with drug misuse, early unnatural death, violent crime, unemployment, homelessness and family violence. Determining the exact nature of the burden associated with antisocial personality disorder is complicated by the definition of the disorder, which conflates impairment (i.e. personality traits) with disability (i.e. antisocial behaviour) and handicap (i.e. adverse social and economic consequences).

In terms of completeness of this epidemiological picture for antisocial personality disorder, there are significant gaps. Comparatively little is known about:

(a) the incidence of the disorder;
(b) its prevalence in primary care, general psychiatric settings, and UK prisons (which have instead concentrated on 'personality disorder');
(c) protective factors; and
(d) the natural history of the disorder.

All of these are potential areas for future research, although perhaps the most important priority should be the accurate determination of natural history. The long-term follow-up of large cohorts of individuals at high risk of developing antisocial personality disorder would facilitate the accurate delineation of:

(a) risk factors;
(b) protective factors; and
(c) a more representative picture of axis I and axis II associations.

Further study of the natural history of the disorder would also have the benefit of indicating:

(a) preventative strategies; and
(b) appropriate treatment interventions, which would pave the way for controlled treatment studies (Dolan & Coid, 1993).

This review has shown that individuals from the following high-risk groups may represent suitable subjects for such longitudinal studies: those with a family history of antisocial behaviour, children with mixed conduct disorder/hyperactivity symptoms, juvenile delinquents, children with an 'under-controlled' temperament, and abused children.

Future natural history studies should correct for the deficiencies of previous longitudinal research and be characterised by:

(a) repeated follow-ups rather than a single follow-up design, in order to provide a more detailed and accurate picture of the course of antisocial personality disorder;
(b) use of psychosocial outcome variables in preference to conviction data, which have been shown to be inaccurate measures of mental state.

Appropriately, the medical profession has largely abandoned the term psychopathy on the grounds that it is pejorative, refers to a heterogeneous group of individuals, and one which is confusingly also a legal term. (The Reed Report took an important step towards reducing some of this confusion by recommending that the term 'psychopathic disorder' should be replaced by 'personality disorder' in the relevant sections of the English Mental Health Act.) Paradoxically, however, literature on the subject continues to proliferate and the Cleckley/Hare model of psychopathy remains a popular one, particularly in North America. Proponents of this model claim empirical support for the term, although some critics interpret this literature as a disguised attempt to study the concept of 'evil' scientifically. Certainly much of the research cited as scientifically validating the Cleckley/Hare model seems to produce rather tautological findings, since the validating criteria are the same as the criteria used to define psychopathy (i.e. 'poor behavioural control', 'irresponsibility', etc.).

Antisocial personality disorder is a contemporary synonym for psychopathy, although it too is problematic as a concept, since it focuses on antisocial behavioural deficits. As a result, the epidemiological literature on antisocial personality disorder is rather circular, with findings of high prevalence rates in populations of prisoners, the homeless and drug-users. Ideally, from a nosological perspective, personality traits (i.e. the fundamental psychological impairment) should be clearly separated from antisocial behaviour (i.e. the associated disability), along the lines suggested by the International Classification of Impairments, Disabilities and Handicaps (World Health Organization, 1980). At worst, a compromise would be for psychiatric epidemiology to adopt a definition that encompasses both personality traits and behaviours associated with an unstable and antisocial lifestyle. The ICD–10 category of dissocial personality disorder is more satisfactory in this regard, although this review has shown that very little literature exists on this entity.

To complicate matters further, there is now considerable evidence to suggest that the current categorical taxonomy for personality disorders (from which the categories of antisocial personality disorder and dissocial personality disorder derive) is inaccurate and should be wholly or at least partially replaced with a dimensional system. This book has reviewed evidence from a number of sources to support this argument. These include the fact that:

(a) the phenotypic features and disability associated with personality disorders are continuously distributed;

(b) normal personality is probably best conceptualised in terms of at least five dimensions, and that measures of these dimensions predict continuous measures of abnormal personality;

(c) mixed categories of personality disorders are the rule rather than the exception.

Therefore there seem to be two distinct priorities for future epidemiological research into people who behave in a consistently antisocial fashion. First, there needs to be a reconsideration of the current taxonomy for personality disorders – only then will there be a robust enough foundation from which to examine personality disturbance in greater detail. It has been suggested that this could be begun by developing a system that allows both categorical and dimensional classifications to coexist (Tyrer, 1994).

Second, epidemiological research should attempt to move away from the current preoccupation with behavioural indices and aim to achieve a more balanced perspective, by adopting measures that accurately reflect *both* the personality *and* behavioural characteristics of people who behave in a repeatedly antisocial fashion. The ICD–10 category of dissocial personality disorder is superior to DSM–IV antisocial personality disorder criteria in this regard, although it is an under-researched category of disorder which merits further attention.

References

ACRES, D. (1975) The after-care of special hospital patients. In *Report of the Committee on Mentally Abnormal Offenders* (Butler Committee), Cmnd 6244, pp. 291–302. London: HMSO.

ALNÆS, R. & TORGERSEN, A. (1988) The relationship between DSM–III symptom disorders and personality disorders in an outpatient population. *Acta Psychiatrica Scandinavica*, **78**, 348–355.

AMERICAN PSYCHIATRIC ASSOCIATION (1980) *Diagnostic and Statistical Manual of Mental Disorders* (3rd edn) (DSM–III). Washington, DC: APA.

—— (1994) *Diagnostic and Statistical Manual of Mental Disorders* (4th edn) (DSM–IV). Washington, DC: APA.

ANDERSEN, H. S., SESTOFT, D., LILLËBACK, T., *et al* (1996) Prevalence of ICD–10 psychiatric morbidity in random samples of prisoners on remand. *International Journal of the Law and Psychiatry*, **19**, 61–74.

ARBOLEDA-FLOREZ, J. & HELLEY, H. L. (1991) Antisocial burnout: an exploratory study. *Bulletin of the American Academy of Psychiatry and the Law*, **19**, 173–183.

BABIAK, P. (1995) When psychopaths go to work: a case study of an industrial psychopath. *Applied Psychological International Review*, **44**, 171–178.

BAILEY, J. & MACCULLOCH, M. (1992) Patterns of reconviction in patients discharged directly to the community from a special hospital: implications for aftercare. *Journal of Forensic Psychiatry*, **3**, 445–461.

BAKER, L. A. (1986) Estimating genetic correlations among discontinuous phenotypes: an analysis of criminal convictions and psychiatric hospital diagnoses in Danish adoptees. *Behavioural Genetics*, **16**, 127–142.

BAKER, R. & HALL, J. N. (1988) REHAB: A new assessment instrument for chronic psychiatric patients. *Schizophrenia Bulletin*, **14**, 97–111.

BARBER, J. P., FRANK, A., WEISS, R. D., *et al* (1996) Prevalence and correlates of personality disorder diagnoses among cocaine-dependent outpatients. *Journal of Personality Disorders*, **10**, 297–311.

BARON, M., GRUEN, R., RAINER, J. D., *et al* (1985) A family study of schizophrenic and normal control probands: implications for the spectrum concept of schizophrenia. *American Journal of Psychiatry*, **142**, 447–455.

BARRETT, J. E., BARRETT, J. A., OXMAN, T. E., *et al* (1988) The prevalence of psychiatric disorders in a primary care practice. *Archives of General Psychiatry*, **45**, 1100–1106.

BEAUTRAIS, A. L., JOYCE, P. R., MULDER, R. T., *et al* (1996) Prevalence and comorbidity of mental disorders in persons making serious suicide attempts: a case–control study. *American Journal of Psychiatry*, **153**, 1009–1039.

BEBBINGTON, P. (1992) Assessing the need for psychiatric treatment at the district level: the role of surveys. In *Measuring Mental Health Needs* (eds G. Thornicroft, C. R. Brewin & J. Wing), pp. 99–117. London: Gaskell.

——, BREWIN, C. R., MARSDEN, L., *et al* (1996) Measuring the need for psychiatric treatment in the general population: the community version of the MRC Needs for Care Assessment. *Psychological Medicine*, **26**, 229–236.

BERRIOS, G. E. (1993) Personality disorders: a conceptual history. In *Personality Disorder Review* (eds P. Tyrer & G. Stein), pp. 17–41. London: Gaskell.

BIRMINGHAM, L., MASON, D. & GRUBIN, D. (1996) Prevalence of mental disorder in remand prisoners: consecutive case study. *British Medical Journal*, **313**, 1521–1524.

BLACK, D. W., BAUMGARD, C. H. & BELL, S. E. (1995*a*) A 16- to 45-year follow-up of 71 men with antisocial personality disorder. *Comprehensive Psychiatry*, **36**, 130–140.

——, —— & —— (1995*b*) The long-term outcome of antisocial personality disorder compared with depression, schizophrenia and surgical conditions. *Bulletin of the American Academy of Psychiatry and the Law*, **23**, 43–52.

BLACKBURN, R. (1971) Personality types among abnormal homicides. *British Journal of Criminology*, **11**, 14–31.

—— (1975) An empirical classification of psychopathic personality. *British Journal of Psychiatry*, **127**, 456–460.

—— (1986) Patterns of personality deviation among violent offenders: replication and extension an empirical taxonomy. *British Journal of Criminology*, **26**, 254–269.

—— (1988) On moral judgements and personality disorders: the myth of psychopathic personality revisited. *British Journal of Psychiatry*, **153**, 505–512.

BLAND, R. C. & ORN, H. (1986) Family violence and psychiatric disorder. *Canadian Journal of Psychiatry*, **31**, 129–137.

——, NEWMAN, S. C. & ORN, H. (1987) Lifetime co-morbidity in a community sample. *Acta Psychiatrica Scandinavica*, **75**, 383–391.

——, ORN, H. & NEWMAN, S. C. (1988*a*) Lifetime prevalence of psychiatric disorders in Edmonton. *Acta Psychiatrica Scandinavica*, **77** (suppl. 338), 24–32.

——, STEBELSKY, G., ORN, H., *et al* (1988*b*) Psychiatric disorders and unemployment in Edmonton. *Acta Psychiatrica Scandinavica*, **77** (suppl. 338), 72–80.

——, NEWMAN, S. C., DYCK, R. J., *et al* (1990) Prevalence of psychiatric disorders and suicide attempts in a prison population. *Canadian Journal of Psychiatry*, **35**, 407–413.

——, ——, ORN, H., *et al* (1993) Epidemiology of pathological gambling in Edmonton. *Canadian Journal of Psychiatry*, **38**, 108–112.

BLUGLASS, R. (1966) *A Psychiatric Study of Scottish Convicted Prisoners*. MD thesis, University of St Andrews, Scotland.

BOHMAN, M. (1978) Some genetic aspects of alcoholism and criminality. A population of adoptees. *Archives of General Psychiatry*, **35**, 267–276.

——, CLONINGER, R., SIGVARDSSON, S., *et al* (1982) Predisposition to petty criminality in Swedish adoptees. Genetic and environmental heterogeneity. *Archives of General Psychiatry*, **39**, 1233–1241.

BOWDEN, P. (1978) Men remanded into custody for medical reports: the selection for treatment. *British Journal of Psychiatry*, **133**, 320–331.

BRADSHAW, J. (1972) A taxonomy of social need. In *Problems and Progress in Medical Care: Essays on Current Research* (ed. G. McLachlan). Oxford: Oxford University Press.

BRAUN, D. L., SUNDAY, S. R. & HALMI, K. A. (1994) Psychiatric comorbidity in patients with eating disorders. *Psychological Medicine*, **24**, 859–867.

BREMER, J. (1951) A social psychiatric investigation of a small community in northern Norway. *Acta Psychiatrica et Neurologica Scandinavica*, suppl. 62.

BREWIN, C. (1992) Measuring individual needs for care and services. In *Measuring Mental Health Needs* (eds G. Thornicroft, C. R. Brewin & J. Wing), pp. 220–236. London: Gaskell.

——, WING, J., MANGEN, S., *et al* (1987) Principles and practice of measuring needs in the long-term mentally ill: the MRC Needs for Care Assessment. *Psychological Medicine*, **17**, 971–981.

—— & —— (1993) The MRC Needs for Care Assessment: progress and controversies. *Psychological Medicine*, **23**, 837–841.

BROOKE, E. M. (1980) Information in mental health services: a tripartite system. *Acta Psychiatrica Scandinavica*, **62** (suppl. 285), 291–297.

BROONER, R. K., GREENFIELD, L., SCHMIDT, C. W., *et al* (1993) Antisocial personality disorder and HIV infection among intravenous drug abusers. *American Journal of Psychiatry*, **150**, 53–58.

——, KING, V. L., KIDORF, M., *et al* (1997) Psychiatric and substance use comorbidity among treatment-seeking opioid abusers. *Archives of General Psychiatry*, **54**, 71–80.

BROTHWELL, J., CASEY, P. & TYRER, P. (1992) Who gives the most reliable account of a patient's personality? *Irish Journal of Psychological Medicine*, **9**, 90–93.

BUCHANAN, A. (1998) Criminal conviction after discharge from special (high security) hospital: incidence in the first 10 years. *British Journal of Psychiatry*, **172**, 472–476.

BUSS, A. H. & PLOMIN, R. (1975) *A Temperamental Theory of Personality*. New York: Wiley.

CADORET, R. J. (1978) Psychopathology in adopted-away offspring of biologic parents with antisocial behaviour. *Archives of General Psychiatry*, **35**, 176–184.

——, O'GORMAN, T. W., TRAUGHTON, E., *et al* (1985) Alcoholism and antisocial personality. *Archives of General Psychiatry*, **42**, 161–167.

CARROLL, K. M., BALL, S. A. & RAINSAVILLE, B. J. (1993) A comparison of alternate systems for diagnosing antisocial personality disorder in cocaine abusers. *Journal of Nervous and Mental Disease*, **181**, 436–443.

CASEY, P. R., DILLON, S. & TYRER, P. (1984) The diagnostic status of patients with conspicuous psychiatric morbidity in primary care. *Psychological Medicine*, **14**, 673–681.

—— & TYRER, P. (1986) Personality, functioning and symptomatology. *Journal of Psychiatric Research*, **20**, 363–374.

—— & —— (1990) Personality disorder and psychiatric illness in general practice. *British Journal of Psychiatry*, **156**, 261–265.

CASPI, A. & SILVA, P. A. (1995) Temperamental qualities at age 3 predict personality traits in young adulthood: longitudinal evidence from a birth cohort. *Child Development*, **66**, 486–498.

——, MOFFITT, T. E., NEWMAN, D. L., *et al* (1996) Behavioural observations at age 3 years predict adult psychiatric disorders. Longitudinal evidence from a birth cohort. *Archives of General Psychiatry*, **53**, 1033–1039.

CHEN, C., WONG, J., LEE, N., *et al* (1993) The Shatin Community Mental Health Survey in Hong Kong. II: Major findings. *Archives of General Psychiatry*, **50**, 125–133.

CHENG, A. T. A., MANN, A. H. & CHAN, K. A. (1997) Personality disorder and suicide. *British Journal of Psychiatry*, **170**, 441–446.

CHESS, S. & THOMAS, A. (1984) *Origins and Evolution of Behaviour Disorders*. New York: Raven Press.

CHILES, J. A., VAN CLEVE, E., JEMELKA, R. P., *et al* (1990) Substance abuse and psychiatric disorders in prison inmates. *Hospital and Community Psychiatry*, **41**, 1132–1133.

CHISWICK, D. (1992) Compulsory treatment of patients with psychopathic disorder: an abnormally aggressive or seriously irresponsible exercise. *Criminal Behaviour and Mental Health*, **2**, 106–113.

CHRISTIANSEN, K. O. (1974) The genesis of aggressive criminality. Implications of a study of crime in a Danish twin study. In *Determinants and Origins of Aggressive Behaviour* (eds J. DeWit & W. W. Hartup). The Hague: Mouton.

CLARK, L. A. (1989) The basic traits of PD: primary and higher-order dimensions. Paper presented at the 97th Convention of the American Psychological Association (unpublished document; available on request from the Division of Mental Health, World Health Organization, 1211 Geneva 27, Switzerland).

CLARKIN, J. F. & KENDALL, P. C. (1992) Comorbidity and treatment planning: summary and future directions. *Journal of Consulting and Clinical Psychology*, **60**, 904–908.

CLECKLEY, H. (1941) *The Mask of Sanity*. St Louis, MO: C. V. Mosby Co.

CLIFFORD, P., CHARMAN, A., WEBB, Y., *et al* (1991) Planning for community care: the Community Placement Questionnaire. *British Journal of Clinical Psychology*, **30**, 193–211.

CLONINGER, C. R. (1978) The antisocial personality. *Hospital Practice*, **13**, 97–106.

—— (1987) *Tridimensional Personality Questionnaire (TPQ)*. Washington, DC: Washington University School of Medicine, Department of Psychiatry and Genetics.

——, REICH, J. & GUZE, J. B. (1975) The multifactorial model of disease transmission II. Sex differences in the familial transmission of sociopathy. *British Journal of Psychiatry,* **127**, 11–22.

——, CHRISTIAN, K. O., REICH, T., *et al* (1978) Implications of sex differences in the prevalence of antisocial personality, alcoholism, and criminality for familial transmission. *Archives of General Psychiatry*, **35**, 1242–1247.

——, SIGVARDSSON, S., BOHMANN, M., *et al* (1982) Predisposition to petty criminality in Swedish adoptees. II: Cross-fostering analysis of gene–environment interaction. *Archives of General Psychiatry*, **39**, 1242–1247.

COID, J. W. (1984) How many psychiatric patients in prison? *British Journal of Psychiatry*, **145**, 78–86.

—— (1988) Mentally abnormal prisoners on remand: I . Rejected or accepted by the NHS? *British Medical Journal*, **296**, 1779–1783.

—— (1992) DSM–III diagnosis in criminal psychopaths: a way forward. *Criminal Behaviour and Mental Health*, **2**, 78–79.

—— (1996) Psychopathology in psychopaths: a study of diagnostic comorbidity and aetiology. MD thesis, University of London.

COMPTON, W. M., HELZER, J. E., HWU, H.-G., *et al* (1991) New methods in cross-cultural psychiatry: psychiatric illness in Taiwan and the United States. *American Journal of Psychiatry*, **148**, 1697–1704.

COOKE, D. J. (1994) *Psychological Disturbance in the Scottish Prison System: Prevalence, Precipitants and Policy*. Scottish Prison Service Occasional Paper No.3. Edinburgh: Scottish Prison Service.

—— (1997) Psychopaths: oversexed, overplayed but not over here? *Criminal Behaviour and Mental Health*, **7**, 3–11.

COOPER, B. (1965) A study of one hundred chronic psychiatric patients identified in general practice. *British Journal of Psychiatry*, **111**, 595–605.

—— (1972) Clinical and social aspects of chronic neurosis. *Proceedings of the Royal Society of Medicine*, **65**, 512–519.

COPE, R. & WARD, M. (1993) What happens to special hospital patients admitted to medium security? *Journal of Forensic Psychiatry*, **4**, 13–24.

CÔTÉ, G. & HODGINS, S. (1990) Co-occurring mental disorders among criminal offenders. *Bulletin of the American Academy of Psychiatry and the Law*, **18**, 271–281.

—— & —— (1992) The prevalence of major mental disorders among homicide offenders. *International Journal of Law and Psychiatry*, **15**, 89–99.

CROWE, R. R. (1972) The adopted offspring of women criminal offenders: a study of their arrest records. *Archives of General Psychiatry*, **27**, 600–603.

CROWELL, J. A., WATERS, E., KRING, A., *et al* (1993) The psychosocial etiologies of personality disorder: what is the answer like? *Journal of Personality Disorders*, suppl. 1, 118–128.

CURRAN, D. & MALLINSON, P. (1944) Psychopathic personality. *Journal of Mental Science*, **90**, 266–286.

—— & PATRIDGE, M. (1963) *Psychological Medicine* (5th edn). London: E. S. Livingstone.

CUTTING, J., COWEN, P. J., MANN, A. H., *et al* (1986) Personality and psychosis: use of the Standardised Assessment of Personality. *Acta Psychiatrica Scandinavica*, **73**, 87–92.

DAHL, A. A. (1986) Some aspects of DSM–III personality disorders illustrated by a consecutive sample of hospitalised patients. *Acta Psychiatrica Scandinavica*, **73** (suppl. 328), 61–66.

DALGAARD, O. S. & KRINGLEN, E. (1976) A Norwegian study of criminality. *British Journal of Criminology*, **16**, 213–232.

DANIEL, A. E., ROBINS, A. J., REID, J. C., *et al* (1988) Lifetime and six-month prevalence of psychiatric disorders among sentenced female offenders. *Bulletin of the American Academy of Psychiatry and the Law*, **16**, 333–342.

DARKE, S., HALL, W. & SWIFT, W. (1994) Prevalence, symptoms and correlates of antisocial personality disorder among methadone maintenance clients. *Drug and Alcohol Dependence*, **34**, 253–257.

DAVIES, W. & FELDMAN, P. (1981) The diagnosis of psychopathy by forensic specialists. *British Journal of Psychiatry*, **138**, 329–331.

DE GIROLAMO, G. & REICH, J. H. (1993) *Personality Disorders*. Geneva: WHO.

DEJONG, L. A. J., VAN DEN BRINK, W., HARTEVELD, F. M., *et al* (1993) Personality disorders in alcoholics and drug addicts. *Comprehensive Psychiatry*, **34**, 87–94.

DELL, S., GROUNDS, A., JAMES, K., *et al* (1991) *Mentally Disordered Remand Prisoners. Report to the Home Office*. London: Home Office.

DEPARTMENT OF HEALTH (1997) *In-patients Formally Detained in Hospitals under the Mental Health Act 1983 and Other Legislation, England: 1990–91 to 1995–96*. Statistical Bulletin 1997/4. London: Department of Health.

—— & HOME OFFICE (1994) *Report of the Department of Health and Home Office Working Group on Psychopathic Disorder*. London: Department of Health.

DICKERSIN, K., SCHERER, E. & LEFEBVRE, C. (1994) Identification of relevant studies for systematic reviews. *British Medical Journal*, **121** (ACP Journal Club Supplement 3), A10–A11.

DIGMAN, J. M. (1990) Personality structure: emergence of the five-factor model. *Annual Review of Psychology*, **41**, 417–440.

DILLING, H., WEYERER, S. & FICHTER, M. (1989) The Upper Bardrian Studies. *Acta Psychiatrica Scandinavica*, **79** (suppl. 348), 113–140.

DINWIDDIE, S. H. (1992) Psychiatric disorders among wife batterers. *Comprehensive Psychiatry*, **33**, 411–416.

——, REICH, T. & CLONINGER, C. R. (1990) Solvent use and psychiatric comorbidity. *British Journal of Addiction*, **85**, 1647–1656.

——, —— & —— (1992) Psychiatric co-morbidity and suicidality among intravenous drug users. *Journal of Clinical Psychiatry*, **53**, 364–369.

—— & BUCHOLZ, K. K. (1993) Psychiatric diagnoses of self-reported child abusers. *Child Abuse and Neglect*, **17**, 465–476.

DOHRENWEND, B. P. & DOHRENWEND, B. S. (1982) Perspectives on the past and future of psychiatric epidemiology (the 1981 Rema Lapouse Lecture). *American Journal of Public Health*, **72**, 1271–1279.

DOLAN, B. & COID, J. W. (1993) *Psychopathic and Antisocial Personality Disorders: Treatment and Research Issues*. London: Gaskell.

—— & MITCHELL, E. (1994) Personality disorder and psychological disturbance of female prisoners: a comparison with women referred for NHS treatment of personality disorder. *Criminal Behaviour and Mental Health*, **4**, 130–143.

——, EVANS, C. & NORTON, K. (1995) Multiple axis II diagnoses of personality disorder. *British Journal of Psychiatry*, **166**, 107–112.

DOLAN, M. (1994) Psychopathy – a neurobiological perspective. *British Journal of Psychiatry*, **165**, 151–159.

DRAKE, R. E. & VAILLANT, G. E. (1988) Longitudinal views of personality disorder. *Journal of Personality Disorders*, **2**, 44–48.

DYCK, R. J., BLAND, R. C., NEWMAN, S. C., *et al* (1988) Suicide attempts and psychiatric disorders in Edmonton. *Acta Psychiatrica Scandinavica*, **77** (suppl. 338), 64–71.

EASTMAN, N. & PEAY, J. (1998) Sentencing psychopaths: is the "Hospital and Limitation Direction" an ill-considered hybrid? *Criminal Law Review*, suppl. (February), 93–108.

ELSE, L., WONDERLICH, S. A., BEATTY, W. W., *et al* (1993) Personality characteristics of men who physically abuse women. *Hospital and Community Psychiatry*, **44**, 54–58.

ENDICOTT, J. & SPITZER, R. L. (1979) Use of the Research Diagnostic Criteria and the Schedule for Affective Disorders and Schizophrenia to study affective disorders. *American Journal of Psychiatry*, **136**, 52–56.

ERONEN, M., HAKOLA, P. & TIIHONEN, J. (1996) Mental disorders and homicidal behaviour in Finland. *Archives of General Psychiatry*, **53**, 497–501.

ESSEN-MOLLER, E. (1956) Individual traits and morbidity in a Swedish rural population. *Acta Psychiatrica et Neurologica Scandinavica*, suppl. 100.

FARAONE, S. V., BIEDERMAN, J., KEENAN, K., *et al* (1991) Separation of DSM–III attention deficit disorder and conduct disorder: evidence from a family-genetic study of American child psychiatric patients. *Psychological Medicine*, **21**, 109–121.

FARRINGTON, D. P. (1986) Age and crime. In *Crime and Justice: An Annual Review of Research*, Vol. 7 (eds M. Tonry & N. Morris), pp. 189–250. Chicago, IL: University of Chicago Press.

—— (1990) Implications of criminal career reasearch for the prevention of offending. *Journal of Adolescence*, **13**, 93–113.

—— (1992) Criminal career research in the United Kingdom. *British Journal of Criminology*, **32**, 521–536.

—— (1993) Childhood origins of teenage antisocial behaviour and adult social dysfunction. *Journal of the Royal Society of Medicine*, **86**, 13–17.

——, GALLAGHER, B., MORLEY, L., *et al* (1988) Are there any successful men from criminogenic backgrounds? *Psychiatry*, **51**, 116-130.

——, LOEBER, R. & VAN KAMMEN, W. (1990) Long term criminal outcomes of hyperactivity-impulsivity-attention deficit and conduct problems in childhood. In *Straight and Devious Pathways from Childhood to Adulthood* (eds L. N. Robins & M. Rutter), pp. 62–81. Cambridge: Cambridge University Press.

—— & WEST, D. J. (1990) The Cambridge Study in Delinquent Development: a long-term follow-up of 411 males. In *Criminality: Personality, Behaviour and Life History* (eds H. J. Kerner & G. Kaiser), pp. 115–138. Berlin: Springer-Verlag.

FAULK, M. (1976) A psychiatric study of men serving a sentence in Winchester Prison. *Medicine, Science and the Law*, **16**, 244–251.

FEIGHNER, J. P., ROBINS, E., GUZE, S. B., *et al* (1972) Diagnostic criteria for use in psychiatric research. *Archives of General Psychiatry*, **26**, 57–63.

FEINSTEIN, A. R. (1970) The pre-therapeutic classification of comorbidity in chronic disease. *Journal of Chronic Diseases*, **23**, 455–468.

FOLSTEIN, M. P., ROMANUSKI, A. J., NESTADT, G., *et al* (1985) Brief report on the clinical reappraisal of the DIS carried out at the Johns Hopkins site of the Epidemiological Catchment Area programme of the NIMH. *Psychological Medicine*, **15**, 809–814.

FRANCES, A. J. (1980) The DSM–III personality disorder section: a commentary. *American Journal of Psychiatry*, **147**, 1439–1448.

FRIEDRICH, W. N. & LUECKE, W. J. (1988) Young school-age sexually aggressive children. *Professional Psychologist: Research and Practice*, **19**, 155–164.

GARMEZY, N. (1981) Personality development. In *Further Explorations in Personality* (eds A. J. Robin, A. M. Aronoff, R. A. Barclay, *et al*), pp. 196–269. New York: Wiley.

GARVEY, M. J. & SPODEN, F. (1980) Suicide attempts in antisocial personality disorder. *Comprehensive Psychiatry*, **21**, 146–149.

GIBBENS, T. C. N., POND, D. A. & STAFFORD-CLARK, D. (1955) A follow-up study of criminal psychopaths. *British Journal of Delinquency*, **6**, 126–136.

GILL, K., NOLIMAL, D. & CROWLEY, T. J. (1992) Antisocial personality disorder, HIV risk behaviour and retention in methadone maintenance therapy. *Drug and Alcohol Dependence*, **30**, 247–252.

GITTELMAN, R., MANNUZZA, S., SHENKER, R., *et al* (1985) Hyperactive boys almost grown up. *Archives of General Psychiatry*, **42**, 937–947.

GLASER, W. F. (1985) Admissions to a prison psychiatric unit. *Australian and New Zealand Journal of Psychiatry*, **19**, 45–52.

GLUEK, B. (1918) A study of 608 admissions to Sing Sing prison. *Mental Hygiene*, **2**, 85–151.

GOLDBERG, D. P. & HUXLEY, P. (1980) *Mental Illness in the Community*. London: Tavistock.

GOODWIN, D. W., SCHULSINGER, F., HERMANSEN, L., *et al* (1973) Alcohol problems in adoptees raised apart from alcoholic biological parents. *Archives of General Psychiatry*, **28**, 238–243.

GROVE, W. M., ECKERT, E. D., HESTON, L., *et al* (1990) Heritability of substance abuse and antisocial behaviour: a study of monozygotic twins reared apart. *Biological Psychiatry*, **27**, 1293–1304.

GUNDERSON, J. G., KOLB, J. & AUSTIN, V. (1981) The Diagnostic Interview for Borderline Patients. *American Journal of Psychiatry*, **138**, 896–903.

—— & PHILLIPS, K. A. (1994) Personality disorders. In *Comprehensive Textbook of Psychiatry* (Vol. 2, 6th edn) (eds H. J. Kaplan & B. J. Sadock), pp. 1425–1463. Baltimore, MD: Williams and Williams.

GUNN, J. & ROBERTSON, G. (1976) Psychopathic personality: a conceptual problem. *Psychological Medicine*, **6**, 631–634.

——, ——, DELL, S., *et al* (1978) *Psychiatric Aspects of Imprisonment*. London: Academic Press.

——, MADEN, T. & SWINTON, M. (1991) *Mentally Disordered Prisoners. Report Commissioned by the Home Office*. London: Home Office.

GUY, E., PLATT, J. J., ZWERLING, I., *et al* (1985) Mental health status of prisoners in an urban jail. *Criminal Justice and Behaviour*, **12**, 29–53.

GUZE, S. B. (1976) *Criminality and Psychiatric Disorders*. New York: Oxford University Press.

——, WOLFGRAM, E. D., McKINNEY, J. K., *et al* (1967) Psychiatric illness in the families of convicted criminals: a study of 519 first-degree relatives. *Diseases of the Nervous System*, **10**, 651–659.

HAMILTON, J. (1990) Special hospitals and the state hospital. In *Principles and Practice of Forensic Psychiatry* (eds R. Bluglass & P. Bowden), pp. 1363–1373. Edinburgh: Churchill Livingstone.

HARE, R. D. (1980) A research scale for the assessment of psychopathy in criminal populations. *Personality and Individual Differences*, **1**, 111–117.

—— (1983) Diagnosis of antisocial personality disorder in two prison populations. *American Journal of Psychiatry*, **140**, 887–890.

—— (1991) *The Hare Psychopathy Checklist – Revised*. Toronto: Multi Health Systems.

—— & JUTAI, J. W. (1983) Criminal history of the male psychopath: Some preliminary data. In *Prospective Studies of Crime and Delinquency* (eds K. T. Van Dusen & S. A. Mednick), pp. 225–236. Boston, MA: Kluwer-Nijhoff.

—— & McPHERSON, L. M. (1994) Violent and aggressive behaviour by criminal psychopaths. *International Journal of Law and Psychiatry*, **7**, 35–50.

—— & HART, S. (1995) Commentary on antisocial personality disorder: the DSM–IV field trial. In *The DSM–IV Personality Disorders* (ed. J. Livesley), pp. 127–134. New York: Guilford Press.

HARPUR, T. J. & HARE, R. D. (1994) Assessment of psychopathy as a function of age. *Journal of Abnormal Psychology*, **103**, 604–609.

HARRIS, G. T., RICE, M. E. & CORMIER, C. A. (1991) Psychopathy and violent recidivism. *Law and Human Behaviour*, **15**, 625–637.

HART, S. D., KROPP, P. R. & HARE, R. D. (1988) Performance of male psychopaths following conditional release from prison. *Journal of Consulting and Clinical Psychology*, **56**, 227–232.

——, DUTTON, D. G. & NEWLOVE, T. (1993) The prevalence of personality disorder among wife assaulters. *Journal of Personality Disorders*, **7**, 329–341.

—— & HARE, R. (1994) Psychopathy and the Big 5: correlations between observers' ratings of normal and pathological personality. *Journal of Personality Disorders*, **8**, 32–40.

HELGASON, T. (1981) Psychiatric epidemiological studies in Iceland. In *Longitudinal Research: Methods and Uses in Behavioural Sciences* (eds F. Schulsinger, S. A. Mednick & J. Knap), pp. 145–155. Boston, MA: Martinus Nijhoff.

HEMPHILL, J. F., HART, S. D. & HARE, R. D. (1994) Psychopathy and substance use. *Journal of Personality Disorders*, **8**, 169–180.

HERMAN, J. L. (1986) Histories of violence in an outpatient population: an exploratory study. *American Journal of Orthopsychiatry*, **56**, 137–141.

HODGINS, S. (1995) Assessing mental disorder in the criminal justice system: feasibility versus clinical accuracy. *International Journal of Law and Psychiatry*, **18**, 15–28.

——, MEDNICK, S. A., BRENNAN, P. A., *et al* (1996) Mental disorder and crime: evidence from a Danish birth cohort. *Archives of General Psychiatry*, **53**, 489–496.

HOFFART, A., THORNES, K., HEDLEY, L.M., *et al* (1994) DSM III-R Axis I and II disorders in agoraphobic patients with and without panic disorder. *Acta Psychiatrica Scandinavica*, **89**, 186–191.

HOGG, L. & MARSHALL, M. (1992) Can we measure need in the homeless mentally ill? Using the MRC Needs for Care Assessment in hostels for the homeless. *Psychological Medicine*, **22**, 1027–1034.

HOLLOWAY, F. (1994) Need in community psychiatry: a consensus is required. *Psychiatric Bulletin*, **18**, 321–323.

HOME OFFICE & DEPARTMENT OF HEALTH AND SOCIAL SERVICES (1975) *Report of the Committee on Mentally Abnormal Offenders*. Cmnd 6244. London: HMSO.

HONDA, Y. (1983) DSM–III in Japan. In *International Perspectives on DSM–III* (eds R. L. Spitzer, J. B. W. Williams & A. E. Skodd), pp. 86–95. Washington, DC: American Psychiatric Press.

HURLEY, W. & DUNNE, P. (1991) Psychological distress and psychiatric morbidity in women prisoners. *Australian and New Zealand Journal of Psychiatry*, **25**, 461–470.

HUESMANN, L. R., ERAN, L. D., LEFKOWITZ, M. M., *et al* (1984) Stability of aggression over time and generations. *Developmental Psychology*, **20**, 1120–1134.

HWU, H. G., YEH, E. K. & CHANG, L. Y. (1989) Prevalence of psychiatric disorders in Taiwan defined by the Chinese Diagnostic Interview Schedule. *Acta Psychiatrica Scandinavica*, **79**, 136–147.

HYLER, S. E. & REIDER, R. O. (1984) *Personality Diagnostic Questionnaire, Revised (PDQ–R)*. New York: New York State Psychiatric Institute.

—— & LYONS, M. (1988) Factor analysis of the DSM–III personality disorder clusters: a replication. *Comprehensive Psychiatry*, **29**, 304–308.

——, RIEDER, R. O., WILLIAMS, J. B. W., *et al* (1989) A comparison of clinical and self-report diagnoses of DSM–III personality disorders in 522 patients. *Comprehensive Psychiatry*, **30**, 170–178.

INTRATOR, J., HARE, R., STRITZKE, P., *et al* (1997) A brain imaging (single photon emission computerised tomography) study of semantic and affective processing in psychopaths. *Biological Psychiatry*, **42**, 96–103.

JACKSON, H. J., WHITESIDE, H. L., BATES, G. W., *et al* (1991) Diagnosing personality disorders in psychiatric inpatients. *Acta Psychiatrica Scandinavica*, **83**, 206–213.

JONES, D. A. (1976) *The Health Risks of Imprisonment*. Lexington, MA: Lexington Books.

JORDAN, K., SCHLENGER, W. E., FAIRBANK, J. A., *et al* (1996) Prevalence of psychiatric disorders among incarcerated women. II: Convicted felons entering prison. *Archives of General Psychiatry*, **53**, 513–519.

KAGAN, J. & MOSS, H. A. (1962) *Birth to Maturity: A Study in Psychological Development*. New York: Wiley.

KASS, F., SKODOL, A. E., CHARLES, E., *et al* (1985) Scaled ratings of DSM–III personality disorders. *American Journal of Psychiatry*, **142**, 627–630.

KESSEL, N. (1960) Psychiatric morbidity in a London general practice. *British Journal of Preventive and Social Medicine*, **14**, 16–22.

KESSLER, L. G., CLEARY, P. D. & BURKE, J. D. (1985) Psychiatric disorders in primary care. *Archives of General Psychiatry*, **42**, 583–587.

KESSLER, R. C., MCGONAGLE, K. A., ZAO, S., *et al* (1994) Lifetime and 12-month prevalence of DSM–III–R psychiatric disorders in the United States: results from the National Comorbidity Survey. *Archives of General Psychiatry*, **51**, 8–19.

——, NELSON, C. B., MCGONAGLE, K. A., *et al* (1996) The epidemiology of co-occurring addictive and mental disorders: implications for prevention and service utilization. *American Journal of Orthopsychiatry*, **66**, 17–31.

KHANTZIAN, E. J. & TREECE, C. (1985) DSM–III diagnosis of narcotic addicts: recent findings. *Archives of General Psychiatry*, **42**, 505–513.

KISH, L. (1965) *Survey Sampling*. Chichester: Wiley.

KLEIN, M. (1985) *Wisconsin Personality Inventory (WISPI)*. Madison, WI: University of Wisconsin, Department of Psychiatry.

KLEINMAN, P. H., MILLER, A. B., MILLMAN, R. B., *et al* (1990) Psychopathology among cocaine abusers entering treatment. *Journal of Nervous and Mental Disease*, **178**, 442–447.

KOCH, J. A. (1891) *Die psychopathischen Minderwertigkeiten*. Ravensburg: Maier.

KOEGEL, P., BURMAN, A. & FARR, R. K. (1988) The prevalence of specific psychiatric disorders among homeless individuals in the inner city of Los Angeles. *Archives of General Psychiatry*, **45**, 1085–1092.

KOENIGSBERG, H. W., KAPLAN, R. D., GILMORE, M. M., *et al* (1985) The relationship between syndrome and personality disorder in DSM–III: experience with 2462 patients. *American Journal of Psychiatry*, **45**, 1085–1092.

KOKKEVI, A. & STEFANIS, C. (1995) Drug abuse and psychiatric comorbidity. *Comprehensive Psychiatry*, **36**, 329–337.

KOLADA, J. L., BLAND, S. C. & NEWMAN, S. C. (1994) Obsessive–compulsive disorder. *Acta Psychiatrica Scandinavica Supplementum*, **376**, 24–35.

KOSTEN, T. R., ROUNSAVILLE, B. J. & KLEBER, H. D. (1982) DSM–III personality disorders in opiate addicts. *Comprehensive Psychiatry*, **23**, 572–581.

KRAEPELIN, E. (1899) *Psychiatrie* (6th edn). Leipzig: Barth.

KRANZLER, H. R., SATEL, S. & APTER, A. (1994) Personality disorders and associated features in cocaine-dependent inpatients. *Comprehensive Psychiatry*, **35**, 335–340.

KRAWIECCKA, M., GOLDBERG, D. & VAUGHN, M. (1977) A standardised psychiatric assessment scale for rating chronic psychotic patients. *Acta Psychiatrica Scandinavica*, **55**, 99-308.

KREITMAN, N. (1993) The principles of psychiatric epidemiology. In *Companion to Psychiatric Studies* (5th edn) (eds R. E. Kendell & A. K. Zealley), pp. 211–225. London: Churchill Livingstone.

KURUOGLU, A. Ç., ARIKAN, Z., VURAL, G., *et al* (1996) Single photon emission computerised tomography in chronic alcoholism. Antisocial personality disorder may be associated with decreased frontal perfusion. *British Journal of Psychiatry*, **169**, 348–354.

LAHEY, B. B., PIACENTINI, J. C., McBURNETT, K., *et al* (1987) Psychopathology in the parents of children with conduct disorder and hyperactivity. *Journal of the American Academy of Child and Adolescent Psychiatry*, **35**, 163–170.

LANGE, J. (1931) *Crime as Destiny*. London: Allen and Unwin.

LANGNER, T. S. & MICHAEL, S. T. (1963) *Life Stress and Mental Health. The Midtown Manhattan Study*. London: Collier, MacMillan.

LEAF, P. J., LIVINGSTON, M. M. & TISCHLER, G. L. (1985) Contact with health professionals for the treatment of psychiatric and emotional problems. *Medical Care*, **23**, 1322–1337.

LEE, C. K., KWAK, Y. S., YAMAMOTO, J., *et al* (1990) Psychiatric epidemiology in Korea, part 1: gender and age differences in Seoul. *Journal of Nervous and Mental Disease*, **178**, 242–252.

LEIGHTON, A. H. (1959) *My Name is Legion: the Stirling County Study of Psychiatric Disorder and Sociocultural Environment*. New York: Basic Books.

LESAGE, A. D., BOYER, R., GRUNBERG, F., *et al* (1994) Suicide and mental disorders: a case-control study of young men. *American Journal of Psychiatry*, **21**, 1063–1068.

LEVAV, I., KOHN, R., DOHRENWEND, B. P., *et al* (1993) An epidemiological study of mental disorders in a 10-year cohort of young adults in Israel. *Psychological Medicine*, **23**, 691–707.

LEWIS, A. (1974) Psychopathic personality: a most elusive category. *Psychological Medicine*, **4**, 133–140.

LILIENFELD, S. O. (1994) Conceptual problems in the assessment of psychopathy. *Clinical Psychology Review*, **14**, 17–38.

——, VAN VALKENBURG, C., LARNTZ, K., *et al* (1986) The relationship of histrionic personality disorder to antisocial personality and somatization disorders. *American Journal of Psychiatry*, **143**, 718–721.

—— & WALDMAN, I. D. (1990) The relation between childhood attention-deficit disorder and adult antisocial behaviour re-examined: the problem of heterogeneity. *Clinical Psychology Review*, **10**, 699–725.

LILIENFIELD, A. M. (1957) Epidemiological methods and influences in studies of non-infectious diseases. *United States Health Services Science Reports*, **2**, 51–60.

LIVESLEY, W. J., JACKSON, D. N. & SCHROEDER, M. L. (1992) Factorial structure of traits delineating personality disorders in clinical and general population samples. *Journal of Abnormal Psychology*, **101**, 432–440.

——, SCHROEDER, M., JACKSON, D. N., *et al* (1994) Categorical distinctions in the study of personality disorder: implications for classification. *Journal of Abnormal Psychology*, **103**, 6–17.

LLOYD, K. R. & WEICH, S. (1997) The epidemiological toolbox in psychiatry: population-based methods in the study of mental disorders. *Current Opinion in Psychiatry*, **10**, 149–152.

LOEBER, R. (1982) The stability of antisocial and delinquent child behaviour: a review. *Child Development*, **53**, 1431–1446.

——, BRINTHAUPT, V. P. & GREEN, S. (1990) Attention deficits, impulsivity, and hyperactivity with or without conduct problems: relationships to delinquency and unique contextual factors. In *Behaviour Disorders of Adolescence: Research, Intervention, and Policy in Clinical and School Settings* (eds R. J. McMahon & R. D. Peters), pp. 39–61. New York: Plenum Press.

LORANGER, A. W., SUSMAN, V. L., OLDHAM, J. M., *et al* (1987) The Personality Disorder Examination: a preliminary report. *Journal of Personality Disorders*, **1**, 1–13.

——, LENZENWEGER, M. F., GARTNER, A. F., *et al* (1991) Trait–state artefacts and the diagnosis of personality disorders. *Archives of General Psychiatry*, **48**, 720–728.

——, SARTORIUS, N. & ANDREOLI, A. (1994) The International Personality Disorder Examination. The World Health Organization/Alcohol, Drug Abuse and Mental Health Administration International Pilot Study of Personality Disorders. *Archives of General Psychiatry*, **51**, 215–224.

LUNTZ, B. K. & WIDOM, C. S. (1994) Antisocial personality disorder in abused and neglected children grown up. *American Journal of Psychiatry*, **151**, 670–674.

LYNAM, D. R. (1996) Early identification of chronic offenders: who is the fledgling psychopath? *Psychological Bulletin*, **120**, 209–234.

MCDONALD, A. S. & DAVEY, G. C. L. (1996) Psychiatric disorders and accidental injury. *Clinical Psychology Review*, **16**, 105–127.

MCFARLANE, A. C. (1988) The International Classification of Impairments, Disabilities and Handicaps: its usefulness in classifying and understanding biopsychosocial phenomena. *Australian and New Zealand Journal of Psychiatry*, **22**, 31–42.

MCGLASHAN, T. H. (1986) The Chestnut Lodge follow-up study: III. Long-term outcome of borderline personalities. *Archives of General Psychiatry*, **43**, 20–30.

MCGUFFIN, P. & GOTTESMAN, I. I. (1984) Genetic influences on normal and abnormal development. In *Child Psychiatry: Modern Approaches* (2nd edn) (eds M. Rutter & L. Hersov), pp. 17–33. London: Blackwell.

—— & THAPAR, A. (1993) The genetics of personality disorder. In *Personality Disorder Revised* (eds P. Tyrer & G. Stein), pp. 42–63. London: Gaskell.

MADDOCKS, P. D. (1970) A five year follow-up of untreated psychopaths. *British Journal of Psychiatry*, **116**, 511–515.

MADEN, A., SWINTON, M. & GUNN, J. (1994) Psychiatric disorder in women serving a prison sentence. *British Journal of Psychiatry*, **164**, 44–54.

——, TAYLOR, C. J. A., BROOKE, D., *et al* (1995) *Mental Disorder in Remand Prisons. Report commissioned by the Home Office Research and Planning Unit on behalf of the Directorate of Health Care*. London: Home Office.

MADEN, T., CURLE, C., MEUX, C., *et al* (1995) *The Treatment and Security Needs of Special Hospital Patients*. London: Whurr.

MAGNUSSON, D. (1988) *Individual Development from an Interactional Perspective: A Longitudinal Study*. Hillsdale, NJ: Lawrence Erlbaum.

MAIER, W., LICHTERMAN, D., KLINGER, T., *et al* (1992) Prevalence of personality disorders (DSM–III–R) in the community. *Journal of Personality Disorders*, **6**, 187–196.

MANN, A. H. (1993) Epidemiology. In *Principles of Social Psychiatry* (eds D. Bhugra & J. Leff), pp. 25–35. Oxford: Blackwell Scientific.

——, JENKINS, R. & BELSEY, E. (1981) The twelve-month outcome of patients with neurotic illness in general practice. *Psychological Medicine*, **11**, 535–550.

MANNUZZA, S., KLEIN, R. G., BESSLER, A., *et al* (1993) Adult outcome of hyperactive boys: educational achievement, occupational rank, and psychiatric status. *Archives of General Psychiatry*, **46**, 565–576.

MARSHALL, M., HOGG, L. I., GATH, D. H., *et al* (1995) The Cardinal Needs Schedule – a modified version of the MRC Needs for Care Assessment Schedule. *Psychological Medicine*, **25**, 605–617.

MARTIN, R. L., CLONINGER, C. R. & GUZE, S. B. (1982) The natural history of somatisation and substance abuse in women criminals: a six year follow-up. *Comprehensive Psychiatry*, **23**, 528–537.

——, ——, ——, *et al* (1985) Mortality in a follow-up of 500 psychiatric outpatients. II: Cause-specific mortality. *Archives of General Psychiatry*, **42**, 58–66.

MASLOW, A. H. (1954) *Motivation and Personality*. New York: Harper & Row.

MATTHEW, G. K. (1971) Measuring need and evaluating services. In *Portfolio for Health. Problems and Progress in Medical Care* (ed. G. McLachlan) (6th series), pp. 21–33. London: Oxford University Press.

MAVISSAKALIAN, M. (1990) The relationship between panic disorder/agoraphobia and personality disorders. *Psychiatric Clinics of North America*, **13**, 661–684.

MBATIA, J. & TYRER, P. (1988) Personality status of dangerous patients at a special hospital. In *Personality Disorders: Diagnosis, Management and Course* (ed. P. Tyrer), pp. 105–111. London: Wright.

MEDNICK, S. A., GABRIELLI, W. F. & HUTCHINGS, B. (1984) Genetic influences in criminal convictions: Evidence from an adoption cohort. *Science*, **224**, 891–894.

MELLSOP, G., VARGHESE, F. T. N., JOSHUA, S., *et al* (1982) Rehability of Axis II of DSM–III. *American Journal of Psychiatry*, **139**, 1360–1361.

MERIKANGAS, K. R. & WEISSMAN, M. N. (1986) Epidemiology of DSM–III axis II personality disorders. In *American Psychiatric Association Annual Review – Vol. 5* (eds A. J. Frances & R. E. Hales), pp. 258–278. Washington, DC: American Psychiatric Press.

MILLON, T. (1982) *Millon Clinical Multiaxial Inventory Manual* (2nd edn). Minnetonka, MN: National Computer Systems.

—— & DAVIS, R. (1995) Conceptions of personality disorders: historical perspectives, the DSMs, and future directions. In *The DSM–IV Personality Disorders* (ed. W. J. Livesley). New York: Guilford Press.

MITCHISON, S., RIX, K. J. B., RENVOIZE, E. B., *et al* (1994) Recorded psychiatric morbidity in a large prison for male remanded and sentenced prisoners. *Medicine, Science and Law*, **34**, 324–331.

MOFFITT, T. E. (1987) Parental mental disorder and offspring criminal behaviour: an adoption study. *Psychiatry*, **50**, 346–360.

—— (1990) Juvenile delinquency and attention deficit disorder: boys developmental trajectories from age 3 to age 15. *Child Development*, **61**, 893–910.

MOLDIN, S. O., RICE, J. P., ERLENMEYER-KIMLING, L., *et al* (1994) Latest structure of DSM–III–R axis II psychopathology in a normal sample. *Journal of Abnormal Psychology*, **103**, 259–266.

MOREY, L. (1988) Personality disorders under DSM-III: an examination of convergence, and internal consistency. *American Journal of Psychiatry*, **145**, 573–577.

MORRIS, J. N. (1957) *Uses of Epidemiology*. Edinburgh: Livingstone.

MORRIS, N. (1974) The failure of imprisonment: toward a punitive philosophy. *Michigan Law Review*, **72**, 302–315.

MORRISON, J. R. (1980) Childhood hyperactivity in an adult psychiatric population: social factors. *Journal of Clinical Psychiatry*, **41**, 40–43.

MULDER, R. T. (1991) Personality disorders in New Zealand hospitals. *Acta Psychiatrica Scandinavica*, **84**, 197–202.

——, WELLS, J. E., JOYCE, P. R., *et al* (1994) Antisocial women. *Journal of Personality Disorders*, **8**, 279–287.

MURPHY, J. M. (1976) Psychiatric labelling in cross-cultural perspective. *Science*, **191**, 1019–1028.

NACE, E. P., DAVIS, C. W. & GASPARI, J. P. (1991) Axis II comorbidity in substance abusers. *American Journal of Psychiatry*, **148**, 118–120.

NAKAO, K., GUNDERSON, J. D., PHILLIPS, K. A., *et al* (1992) Functional impairment in personality disorders. *Journal of Personality Disorders*, **6**, 24–33.

NARROW, W. E., REGIER, D. A., RAE, D. S., *et al* (1993) Use of services by persons with mental and addictive disorders. Findings from the NIMH ECA program. *Archives of General Psychiatry*, **50**, 95–107.

NESTADT, G., ROMANOSKI, A. J., SAMUELS, J. F., *et al* (1992) The relationship between personality and DSM–III axis I disorders in the population: results from an epidemiological survey. *American Journal of Psychiatry*, **149**, 1228–1233.

NEWMAN, D. L., MOFFITT, T. E., CASPI, A., *et al* (1996) Psychiatric disorder in a birth cohort of young adults: prevalence, comorbidity, clinical significance, and new case incidence from ages 11 to 21. *Journal of Consulting and Clinical Psychology*, **64**, 552–562.

OLDHAM, J. H. (1994) Personality disorders: current perspectives. *Journal of the American Medical Association*, **272**, 1770–1777.

—, SKODOL, A. E., KELLMAN, D., *et al* (1992) Diagnosis of DSM–III–R personality disorders by two structured interviews: patterns of comorbidity. *American Journal of Psychiatry*, **149**, 213–220.

—, —, —, *et al* (1995) Diagnosis of DSM–III–R personality disorders by two structured interviews: pattern of comorbidity. *American Journal of Psychiatry*, **149**, 213–220.

OLIVER, J. E. (1988) Successive generations of child maltreatment: the children. *British Journal of Psychiatry*, **153**, 543–553.

OLWEUS, D. (1977) Aggression and peer acceptance in adolescent boys: two short-term longitudinal studies of ratings. *Child Development*, **48**, 1301–1313.

— (1978) *Aggression in the Schools: Bullies and Whipping Boys*. Washington, DC: Hemisphere.

— (1979) Stability of aggressive reaction patterns in males: a review. *Psychological Bulletin*, **86**, 852–875.

PARIS, J. (1992) Social risk factors for borderline personality disorder: a review and hypothesis. *Canadian Journal of Psychiatry*, **37**, 510–515.

— (1997a) *Social Factors in the Personality Disorders. A Biopsychosocial Approach to Etiology and Treatment*. Cambridge: Cambridge University Press.

— (1997b) Antisocial and borderline personality disorders: two aspects of the same psychopathology. *Comprehensive Psychiatry*, **38**, 237–242.

PATIENCE, D. A., McGUIRE, R. J., SCOTT, A. I. F., *et al* (1995) The Edinburgh Primary Care Depression Study: personality disorder and outcome. *British Journal of Psychiatry*, **167**, 324–330.

PATTERSON, G. R. (1982) *Coercive Family Process*. Eugene, OR: Castalia.

PEPPER, C. M., KLEIN, D. N., ANDERSON, R. S., *et al* (1995) DSM–III–R axis II comorbidity in dysthymia and major depression. *American Journal of Psychiatry*, **152**, 239–247.

PERRY, J. C. (1992) Problems and considerations in the valid assessment of personality disorders. *American Journal of Psychiatry*, **149**, 1645–1653.

— (1993) Longitudinal studies of personality disorders. *Journal of Personality Disorders*, Spring suppl., 63–85.

—, LAVORI, P. W. & HOKE, L. (1985) A Markov model for predicting levels of psychiatric service use in borderline and antisocial personality disorders and bipolar type II affective disorder. *Journal of Psychiatric Research*, **21**, 215–232.

—, —, COOPER, S. H., *et al* (1987) The Diagnostic Interview Schedule and DSM–III antisocial personality disorder. *Journal of Personality Disorders*, **1**, 121–131.

PFOHL, B., STANGL, D. & ZIMMERMAN, M. (1983) *Structured Interview for DSM–III Personality Disorders (SIPD)*. Iowa, IA: University of Iowa.

—, CORYELL, W., ZIMMERMAN, M., *et al* (1986) DSM–III personality disorders: diagnostic overlap and internal consistency of individual DSM–III criteria. *Comprehensive Psychiatry*, **27**, 21–34.

PHELAN, M., SLADE, M., THORNICROFT, G., *et al* (1995) The Camberwell Assessment of Need: the validity and reliability of an instrument to assess the needs of people with severe mental illness. *British Journal of Psychiatry*, **167**, 589–595.

PILGRIM, J. & MANN, A. (1990) Use of the ICD–10 version of the Standardised Assessment of Personality to determine the prevalence of personality disorder in psychiatric in-patients. *Psychological Medicine*, **20**, 985–992.

PLOMIN, R., DeFRIES, J. C. & FULKER, D. W. (1988) *Nature and Nurture During Infancy and Early Childhood.* Cambridge: Cambridge University Press.

POLLOCK, V. E., BRIERE, J., SCHNEIDER, L., *et al* (1990) Childhood antecedents of antisocial behaviour: parental alcoholism and physical abusiveness. *American Journal of Psychiatry*, **147**, 1290–1293.

REGIER, D. A., FARMER, M. E., RAE, D. S., *et al* (1990) Comorbidity of mental health disorders with alcohol and other drug abuse. *Journal of the American Medical Association*, **264**, 2511–2518.

REICH, J. H. & NOYES, R. (1987) A comparison of DSM–III personality disorders in acutely ill panic and depressed patients. *Journal of Anxiety Disorder*, **1**, 123–131.

——, YATES, W. & NDUAGUBA, M. (1989) Prevalence of DSM–III personality disorders in the community. *Social Psychiatry*, **24**, 12–16.

—— & VASILE, R. G. (1993) Effect of personality disorders on the treatment outcome of axis I conditions: an update. *Journal of Nervous and Mental Disease*, **181**, 475–484.

REISS, D., GRUBIN, D. & MEUX, C. (1996) Young 'psychopaths' in special hospital: treatment and outcome. *British Journal of Psychiatry*, **168**, 99–104.

RENNEBERG, B., CHAMBLESS, D. L. & GRACELEY, E. J. (1992) Prevalence of SCID-diagnosed personality disorders in agoraphobic outpatients. *Journal of Anxiety Disorder,* **6**, 111–118.

RICE, M. E., HARRIS, G. T. & QUINSEY, V. L. (1990) A follow-up of rapists assessed in a maximum security psychiatric facility. *Journal of Interpersonal Violence*, **5**, 435–448.

—— & —— (1995) Psychopathy, schizophrenia, alcohol abuse and violent recidivism. *International Journal of Law and Psychiatry*, **18**, 333–342.

ROBERTSON, G. (1989) Treatment of offender patients: how should success be measured? *Medicine, Science and Law*, **29**, 303–307.

ROBERTSON, R. G. (1987) The female offender: a Canadian study. *Canadian Journal of Psychiatry*, **32**, 749–755.

ROBINS, E. & GUZE, S. B. (1970) Establishment of diagnostic validity in psychiatric illness: its application to schizophrenia. *American Journal of Psychiatry*, **126**, 983–987.

ROBINS, L. N. (1966) *Deviant Children Grown Up.* Baltimore, MD: Williams and Wilkins.

—— (1978) Sturdy childhood predictors of adult antisocial behaviour: replications from longitudinal studies. *Psychological Medicine*, **8**, 611–622.

—— (1985) Epidemiology of antisocial personality. In *Psychiatry (vol. 3).* Philadelphia, PA: Lippincott.

—— (1991) Conduct disorder. *Journal of Child Psychology and Psychiatry*, **32**, 193–212.

—— (1995) Commentary on antisocial personality disorder. In *The DSM–IV Personality Disorders* (ed. J. Livesley), pp. 135–140. New York: Guilford Press.

——, HELZER, J. E., CRAIGHAN, J., *et al* (1981) NIMH Diagnostic Interview Schedule. *Archives of General Psychiatry*, **38**, 381–389.

——, Tipp, J., Przybeck, T. (1991) Antisocial personality. In *Psychiatric Disorders in America* (eds L. N. Robins & D. A. Regier), pp. 258–280. New York: Free Press.

—— & REGIER, D. A. (1991) *Psychiatric Disorders in America. The ECA Study.* New York: Free Press.

ROFF, J. D. & WIRT, R. D. (1984) Childhood aggression and social adjustment as antecedents of delinquency. *Journal of Abnormal Child Psychology*, **12**, 111–126.

ROPER, W. F. (1950) A comparative study of the Wakefield Prison population in 1948. Part I. *British Journal of Delinquency*, **1**, 15–28.

—— (1951) A comparative study of the Wakefield Prison population in 1948 and 1949. Part II. *British Journal of Delinquency*, **1**, 243–270.

Ross, H. E. (1995) DSM–III–R alcohol abuse and dependence and psychiatric comorbidity in Ontario: results from the Mental Health Supplement to the Ontario Health Survey. *Drug and Alcohol Dependence*, **39**, 111–128.

Rounsaville, B. J. & Kleber, H. D. (1985) Untreated opiate addicts: how do they differ from those seeking treatment? *Archives of General Psychiatry*, **42**, 1072–1077.

—, Kosten, T. R., Weissman, M. M., *et al* (1986) Prognostic significance of psychiatric disorders among treated opiate addicts. *Archives of General Psychiatry*, **43**, 739–745.

—, Anton, S. F., Carroll, K., *et al* (1991) Psychiatric diagnoses of treatment-seeking cocaine abusers. *Archives of General Psychiatry*, **48**, 43–51.

Rutter, M., Cox, A., Tupling, C., *et al* (1975) Attainment and adjustment in two geographical areas. I: The prevalence of psychiatric disorder. *British Journal of Psychiatry*, **126**, 493–509.

Rydelius, P. A. (1988) The development of antisocial behaviour and sudden violent death. *Acta Psychiatrica Scandinavica*, **77**, 398–403.

Saarento, O., Nieminten, P., Hakko, H., *et al* (1997) Utilization of psychiatric in-patient care among new patients in a comprehensive community-care system: a 3-year follow-up study. *Acta Psychiatrica Scandinavica*, **95**, 132–139.

Samuels, J. F., Nestadt, G., Ramanoski, A. J., *et al* (1994) DSM–III personality disorders in the community. *American Journal of Psychiatry*, **151**, 1055–1062.

Sanderson, W. C., Wetzler, S., Beck, A. T., *et al* (1992) Prevalence of personality disorders in patients with major depression and dysthymia. *Psychiatry Research*, **42**, 93–99.

Sara, G., Raven, P. & Mann, A. (1996) A comparison of DSM–III–R and ICD–10 personality disorder criteria in an out-patient population. *Psychological Medicine*, **26**, 151–160.

Sartorius, N., Üstün, B., Costa E Silva, J.-A., *et al* (1993) An international study of psychological problems in primary care: preliminary report from the WHO collaborative project on 'Psychological Problems in General Health Care'. *Archives of General Psychiatry*, **50**, 819–824.

Sato, T. & Takeichi, M. (1993) Lifetime prevalence of specific psychiatric disorders in a general medical clinic. *General Hospital Psychiatry*, **15**, 224–233.

Schneider, K. (1950) *Die psychopatischen Personlichkeiten*. Vienna: Deuticke.

Schulberg, H. C., Saul, M., McClelland, M., *et al* (1985) Assessing depression in primary medical and psychiatric practices. *Archives of General Psychiatry*, **42**, 1164–1170.

Shiell, A., Gerard, K. & Donaldson, C. (1987) Cost of illness studies: an aid to decision-making? *Health Policy*, **8**, 320–323.

Siever, L. J. & Davis, K. L. (1991) A psychobiological perspective on the personality disorders. *American Journal of Psychiatry*, **148**, 1647–1658.

Sigvardsson, D., Cloninger, C. R., Bohman, M., *et al* (1982) Predisposition to petty criminality in Swedish adoptees: III. Sex differences and the male typology. *Archives of General Psychiatry*, **39**, 1248–1253.

Simonsen, E. & Mellergard, M. (1988) Trends in the use of the borderline diagnosis in Denmark from 1975 to 1985. *Journal of Personality Disorders*, **2**, 102–108.

Skodol, A. E., Oldham, J. M., Rosnick, L., *et al* (1991) Diagnosis of DSM–III–R personality disorders: a comparison of two structured interviews. *Methods in Psychiatric Research*, **1**, 13–26.

Slade, M. & Thornicroft, G. (1995) Health and social needs of the long-term mentally ill. *Current Opinions in Psychiatry*, **8**, 126–129.

Smith, G. R., Golding, J. M., Kashner, M., *et al* (1991) Antisocial personality disorder in primary care patients with somatisation disorder. *Comprehensive Psychiatry*, **32**, 367–372.

Smith, K., Shah, A., Wright, K., *et al* (1995) The prevalence and costs of psychiatric disorders and learning disabilities. *British Journal of Psychiatry*, **166**, 9–18.

Smith, S. S. & Newman, J. P. (1990) Alcohol and drug abuse – dependence in psychopathic and non-psychopathic criminal offenders. *Journal of Abnormal Psychology*, **99**, 430–439.

Soloff, P. H. & Millward, J. W. (1983) Developmental histories of borderline patients. *Comprehensive Psychiatry*, **24**, 574–588.

Special Hospitals Service Authority (1995) *Service Strategies for Secure Care*. London: Special Hospitals Service Authority.

SPITZER, R. L. & WILLIAMS, J. B. W. (1987) *Structured Clinical Interview for DSM–III–R Personality Disorders (SCID–II)*. New York: New York State Psychiatric Institute, Biometric Research Department.

STEELS, M., RONEY, G., LARKIN, E., *et al* (1998) Discharge from special hospital: a comparison of the fates of psychopaths and the mentally ill. *Criminal Behaviour and Mental Health*, **8**, 39–55.

STEVENS, A. & GABBAY, J. (1991) Needs assessment needs assessment. *Health Trends*, **23**, 20–23.

STEWART, M. A., DEBLOIS, C. S. & CUMMINGS, C. (1980) Psychiatric disorder in the parents of hyperactive boys and those with conduct disorder. *Journal of Child Psychology and Psychiatry*, **21**, 283–292.

STONE, M. H. (1993) Long-term outcome in personality disorders. *British Journal of Psychiatry*, **162**, 299–313.

——, HURT, S. W. & STONE, D. K. (1987) The PI-500: long-term follow-up of borderline in-patients meeting DSM–III criteria: I. Global outcome. *Journal of Personality Disorders*, **1**, 291–298.

STORM-MATHISEN, A. & VAGLUM, P. (1994) Conduct disorder patients 20 years later: a personal follow-up study. *Acta Psychiatrica Scandinavica*, **89**, 416–420.

STRAUSS, J. S., HAFEZ, H., LIEBERMAN, P., *et al* (1985) The course of psychiatric disorder, III: longitudinal principles. *American Journal of Psychiatry*, **142**, 289–296.

STROMGREN, E. (1950) Statistical and genetical population studies within psychiatry: methods and principal results. In *Congres International de Psychiatrie Paris VI. Psychiatrie Sociale*, pp. 155–188. Paris: Hermann *et Cie*.

SWANSON, M. C. J., BLAND, R. C. & NEWMAN, S. C. (1994) Antisocial personality disorders. *Acta Psychiatrica Scandinavica*, **376**, 63–70.

SWINTON, M., MADEN, A. & GUNN, J. (1994) Psychiatric disorder in life-sentenced prisoners. *Criminal Behaviour and Mental Health*, **4**, 10–20.

TAYLOR, P. J. (1986) Psychiatric disorders in London's life-sentenced offenders. *British Journal of Criminology*, **26**, 63–78.

—— (1992) *Criminal Behaviour and Mental Health: Special Supplement*, **2**, iii–v.

—— & GUNN, J. (1984) Violence and psychosis. I: Risk of violence among psychotic men. *British Medical Journal*, **288**, 1945–1949.

—— & PARROTT, J. M. (1988) Elderly offenders: a study of age-related factors among custodially remanded prisoners. *British Journal of Psychiatry*, **152**, 340–346.

TENNENT, G. & WAY, C. (1984) The English special hospital – a 12–17 year follow-up study: a comparison of violent and non-violent re-offenders. *Medicine, Science and the Law*, **24**, 81–91.

TEPLIN, L. A., ABRAM, K. M. & MCCLELLAND, G. M. (1996) Prevalence of psychiatric disorders among incarcerated women. I: Pretrial jail detainees. *Archives of General Psychiatry*, **53**, 505–512.

THAPAR, A. & MCGUFFIN, P. (1996) A twin study of antisocial and neurotic symptoms in childhood. *Psychological Medicine*, **26**, 1111–1118.

THOMPSON, A. H. & BLAND, R. C. (1995) Social dysfunction and mental illness in a community sample. *Canadian Journal of Psychiatry*, **40**, 15–20.

THORNICROFT, G., PHELAN, M. & STRATHDEE, G. (1996) Needs assessment. In *Mental Health Service Evaluation* (eds H. Knudsen & G. Thornicroft), pp. 317–338. Cambridge: Cambridge University Press.

TOMASSON, K. & VAGLUM, P. (1995) A nationwide representative sample of treatment-seeking alcoholics: a study of psychiatric comorbidity. *Acta Psychiatrica Scandinavica*, **92**, 378–385.

TYRER, P. (1995) Are personality disorders well classified in DSM–IV? In *The DSM–IV Personality Disorders* (ed. J. Livesley), pp. 29–42. New York: Guilford Press.

—— (1996) Comorbidity or consanguinity. *British Journal of Psychiatry*, **168**, 669–671.

——, CICCHETTI, A. D., COHEN, M. S., *et al* (1979) Reliability of a schedule for rating personality disorders. *British Journal of Psychiatry*, **135**, 168–174.

UNIVERSITY OF YORK (1996) *Undertaking Systematic Reviews of Research on Effectiveness. CRD Guidelines for Those Carrying Out or Commissioning Reviews.* CRD Report No.4. York: NHS Centre for Reviews and Dissemination, University of York.

VIZE, C. & TYRER, P. (1994) The relationship between personality and other psychiatric disorders. *Current Opinion in Psychiatry,* **7**, 123–128.

WALKER, J. L., LAHEY, B. B., HYND, G. W., *et al* (1987) Comparison of specific patterns of antisocial behaviour in children with conduct disorder with or without coexisting hyperactivity. *Journal of Consulting and Clinical Psychology,* **55**, 910–913.

WALKER, M. & McCABE, S. (1973) *Crime and Insanity in England,* Vol.2. Edinburgh: Edinburgh University Press.

WALTERS, G. D. (1990) *The Criminal Lifestyle: Patterns of Serious Criminal Conduct.* Newbury Park, CA: Sage.

WATT, F., TOMISON, A. & TORPY, D. (1993) The prevalence of psychiatric disorder in a male remand population: a pilot study. *Journal of Forensic Psychiatry,* **4**, 75–83.

WEISS, G. & HECHTMAN, L. T. (1986) *Hyperactive Children Grown Up.* New York: Guilford Press.

WEISS, R. D. & MIRIN, S. M. (1986) Subtypes of cocaine abusers. *Psychiatric Clinics of North America,* **9**, 491-501.

——, ——, GRIFFIN, M. C., *et al* (1993) Personality disorders in cocaine dependence. *Comprehensive Psychiatry,* **34**, 145–149.

WEISSMAN, M. M. & MYERS, J. K. (1980) Psychiatric disorders in a US community. *Acta Psychiatrica Scandinavica,* **62**, 99–111.

WELFORD, C. F. (1973) Age composition and the increase in recorded crime. *Criminology,* **11**, 61.

WELLS, J. E., BUSHNELL, J. A., HORNBLOW, A. R., *et al* (1989) Christchurch Psychiatric Epidemiological Study, Part 1: Methodology and lifetime prevalence for specific psychiatric disorders. *Australian and New Zealand Journal of Psychiatry,* **23**, 315–326.

WERNER, E. E. & SMITH, R. S. (1982) *Vulnerable but Invincible: A Study of Resilient Children.* New York: McGraw-Hill.

WEST, D. J. (1969) *Present Conduct and Future Delinquency.* London: Heinemann.

—— (1982) *Delinquency: Its Roots, Careers and Prospects.* London: Heinemann.

—— & FARRINGTON, D. P. (1973) *Who Becomes Delinquent?* London: Heinemann.

—— & —— (1977) *The Delinquent Way of Life.* London: Heinemann.

WIDIGER, T. A. (1987) *Personality Interview Questions II (PIQ–II).* Lexington, KY: University of Kentucky.

——, SANDERSON, C. & WARNER, L. (1986) The MMPI, prototypal typology, and borderline personality disorder. *Journal of Personality Assessment,* **50**, 540–553.

——, TRULL, T., HURT, S., *et al* (1987) A multidimensional sealing of the DSM–III personality disorders. *Archives of General Psychiatry,* **44**, 557–563.

——, ——, HARRIS, M., *et al* (1991) Comorbidity among Axis II disorders . In *Personality Disorders: New Perspectives on Diagnostic Validity* (ed. J. Oldham), pp. 163–194. Washington, DC: American Psychiatric Press.

—— & CORBITT, E. M. (1995) Antisocial personality disorder. In *The DSM–IV Personality Disorders* (ed. J. Livesley), pp. 103–126. New York: Guilford Press.

——, CADORET, R., HARE, R., *et al* (1996) DSM–IV antisocial personality disorder field trial. *Journal of Abnormal Psychology,* **105**, 3–16.

WIDOM, C. S. (1989) The cycle of violence. *Science,* **244**, 160–166.

WIGGINS, J. S. & PINCUS, A. L. (1989) Conceptions of personality disorder and dimensions of personality. *Psychological Assessment,* **1**, 305–316.

WITTCHEN, H.-V. (1996) Critical issues in the evaluation of comorbidity of psychiatric disorders. *British Journal of Psychiatry,* **168** (suppl. 30), 9–16.

——, ROBINS, L. N., COTTLER, L. B., *et al* (1991) Participants in the multicentre WHO/ADAMHA field trials. Cross-cultural feasibility, reliability and sources of variance in the Composite International Diagnostic Interview (CIDI). *British Journal of Psychiatry,* **159**, 645–653.

WOLFF, S. (1993) Personality disorder in childhood. In *Personality Disorder Reviewed* (eds P. Tyrer & G. Stein), pp. 64–89. London: Gaskell.

WOLKIND, S. & RUTTER, M. (1985) Separation, loss and family relationships. In *Child and Adolescent Psychiatry: Modern Approaches* (eds M. Rutter & L. Hersov), pp. 34–57. Oxford: Blackwell.

WOODRUFF, R. A., GUZE, S. G. & CLAYTON, P. J. (1971) The medical and psychiatric implications of antisocial personality (sociopathy). *Diseases of the Nervous System*, **32**, 712–714.

WOODY, G. E., MCLELLAN, A. T., LUBORSKY, L., *et al* (1985) Sociopathy and psychotherapy outcome. *Archives of General Psychiatry*, **42**, 505–513.

WORLD HEALTH ORGANIZATION (1980) *International Classification of Impairments, Disabilities, and Handicaps: A Manual of Classification Relating to the Consequences of Disease*. Geneva: WHO.

—— (1992) *The ICD–10 Classification of Mental and Behavioural Disorders: Clinical Descriptions and Diagnostic Guidelines*. Geneva: WHO.

WYKES, T. & STURT, E. (1986) The measurement of social behaviour in psychiatric patients: an assessment of the reliability and validity of the SBS Schedule. *British Journal of Psychiatry*, **148**, 1–11.

ZANARINI, M. C. (1983) *Diagnostic Interview for Personality Disorders (DIPD)*. Belmont, MA: McLean Hospital, Psychosocial Research Program.

ZEILLER, B. (1982) Physical and psychological abuse: a follow-up of abused delinquent adolescents. *Child Abuse and Neglect*, **6**, 207–210.

ZIMMERMAN, M. (1994) Diagnosing personality disorders: a review of issues and research methods. *Archives of General Psychiatry*, **51**, 225–245.

—— & CORYELL, W. H. (1989) DSM–III personality disorder diagnoses in a non-patient sample. *Archives of General Psychiatry*, **46**, 682–689.

—— & —— (1990) Diagnosing personality disorders in the community. *Archives of General Psychiatry*, **47**, 527–531.

ZOCCOLILLO, M., PICKLES, A., QUINTON, D., *et al* (1992) The outcome of childhood conduct disorder: implications for defining adult personality disorder and conduct disorder. *Psychological Medicine*, **22**, 971–986.

Index

Compiled by LINDA ENGLISH

abuse/neglect in childhood 81, 82–83, 101
adolescents, needs assessment for 97–98
adoption studies 72–74
age differences 18, 50–52
aggression 59, 80–81, 84, 88
alcohol misuse 17, 60, 62, 63, 67, 73–74, 83, 86
anxiety disorder 61, 68, 75
assessment of personality disorders, problems in 2–6
associated conditions, studies of 2, 25, 33, 38, 55–69, 101
    axis I conditions 2–3, 58–68
    axis II conditions 55–58
    studies examining clusters of axis II disorders and/or groups of clinical syndromes 60–61
    studies examining full range of axis I and II disorders 59–60
    studies examining specific categories of axis I disorder 61–68
axis I conditions, co-occurrence with axis II conditions 2–3, 58–68, 101
axis II conditions 6, 7, 8
    and childhood experiences 81–82
    co-occurrence of 55–58, 102
    co-occurrence with axis I conditions 2–3, 58–68, 101
    see also personality disorders

behaviour-based approach to psychopathy xiii–xv
borderline personality disorder 25, 50, 52, 75
    health service utilisation 89
    in prisons/special hospitals 34–35, 39, 40
    relationship with antisocial personality disorder xvi, 28, 58, 59
Briquet's syndrome 70
bulimia 60
burden studies 2, 85–90
'burn-out' 50–52

Camberwell Assessment of Need (CAN) 95–96
Camberwell Assessment of Need, Forensic Version (CAN–F) 96
Cardinal Needs Schedule 95, 97–98
carer stress criterion 95
case definition 13–14
categorical approach to personality disorders 7, 8, 56, 102
chaotic lifestyle as sampling problem 15
child abuse 82–83, 86
childhood
    antecedents of antisocial personality disorder 44–45, 74–84, 101
    prospective studies of 'deviance' 74–79
    studies of temperament 79–81
    traumatic experiences 81–84
    twin studies 72

child-rearing 78, 79, 81–84
classification of personality
  disorders, problems in 6–9
Cleckley/Hare model of
  psychopathy xii, 101
clinical syndromes, co-occurrence
  with 2–3, 58–68
cluster B disorders 60, 68, 72
community surveys 10–20, 63
  demographic correlates 18–20
  main findings 17–18
  methodological considerations
    13–16
comorbidity 2–3, 25, 33, 38,
  55–69, 101
comparative need 91–92
Composite International
  Diagnostic Interview (CIDI) 14
conduct disorders of childhood
  44, 74–77, 84, 101
cooperation criterion 95
cost of illness studies 89–90
Crime (Sentences) Act 1997 viii
criminality
  and 'over-inclusiveness' problem
    xiv
  as outcome measure 43–44, 45,
    50, 51, 74, 101
  as social burden 86–88
  childhood antecedents 77–81, 83
  family studies 70–71
  genetic studies 71, 72–73
  needs assessment of mentally
    disordered offenders and
    psychopaths 34, 38–41, 96–99
  studies in prison settings 28–39,
    67, 92, 98, 100
  studies in special/high security
    hospitals 39–42
cross-cultural differences 17, 24, 33
cycle of violence 82–83

delinquency 101
  studies of development of
    77–79, 80
  twin studies 71

demographic correlates 18–20
depression 60, 68
descriptive studies 1, 10–42
  community surveys 10–20, 63
  studies in primary care 20–24
  studies in prison settings 28–39,
    67, 92, 98, 100
  studies in psychiatric settings
    24–28
  studies in special/high security
    hospitals 39–42
diagnostic equivalents ix
Diagnostic Interview Schedule
  (DIS) 10, 13–14, 16, 33
*Diagnostic and Statistical Manual of
  Mental Disorders*
    antisocial personality disorder
      category x–xi, xii, xiii–xv, 2,
      33
    DSM–III 7, 33, 58, 62
    DSM–IV x–xi, xii, xiii–xv, 2,
      43, 55, 62
    see also axis I *and* axis II
      conditions
dimensional approach to
  personality disorders 7–8,
  102
disability 85, 100, 102
dissocial personality disorder ix,
  xi, xiii, xiv–xv, xvi, 21, 53, 102,
  103
divorce 86
drop-out bias 50
drug misuse xiv, 33, 60, 61, 62–67,
  86, 89, 98
dysphoric affect 62
dysthymia 60

eating disorders 60, 61, 68
economic burden 89–90
educational status 19, 78, 79
Epidemiological Catchment Area
  (ECA) study 15, 16, 19, 63
explosive personality disorder 21,
  27
expressed need 91

family studies 70–71, 77, 80
felt need 91
finished consultant episodes 27–28
first-generation studies 11
five-factor model of personality
    7–8
fledgling psychopaths 77
fourth generation studies, need
    for 93
friendships 79

gambling 68
gender biases 3
gender differences 18, 71
genetic studies 70–74, 77

handicap 85, 100
health service utilisation 88–90, 93
high security hospitals, studies in
    39–42
histrionic personality disorder 3,
    27, 58
HIV risk-taking behaviour 66–67
homelessness 15, 86, 98
homicide 33, 88
hospital admission data 27–28,
    41–42
hyperactivity, childhood 76–77,
    101
hysteria 70

impaired recall problem 16
impairment 85, 93, 100, 102
impulsivity 59, 79, 80
incidence studies 10, 100
inhibited temperament 80, 81
*International Classification of
    Diseases* (ICD–10) xi, xiii, xiv–xv,
    21, 43, 59, 102, 103
*International Classification of
    Impairments, Disabilities and
    Handicaps* 85, 102
International Personality Disorder
    Examination 3
intravenous drug use 66
Israel 17–18, 20

Japan 24
juvenile delinquency 101
    studies of development of
        77–79, 80
    twin studies 71

Kish method 16

lifetime prevalence, use of 16
longitudinal studies
    see natural history studies

mania 60
marital status 19
medical need/demand/utilisation
    92
Mental Health Act 1983 xi, 41, 42
mental health service usage 88–90
mentally disordered offenders and
    needs assessment 34, 38–39,
    40–41, 96–99
Minnesota Multiphasic Personality
    Inventory (MMPI) 8
mixed conduct disorder/
    hyperactivity symptoms 76–77,
    101
mood disorder 61
MRC Needs for Care Assessment
    93–95, 99

narcissistic personality disorder 58
National Comorbidity Survey 19,
    63, 67–68
natural history studies 1, 43–54,
    100–101
    antisocial 'burn-out' 50–52
    conclusions from longitudinal
        studies 54
    literature search findings
        44–50
    methodological
        considerations 43–44
    suicide 52–54
need/demand/supply distinction
    92
needle-sharing 66–67

needs assessment 91–99
  defining need 91–92, 93, 98
  individual 93–96
  measurement of need 92–99
  of mentally disordered
    offenders and psychopaths 34,
    38–39, 40–41, 96–99
  population-based 92–93
NHS and Community Care Act
  1990 91, 95
non-response problem 15, 39
normal personality traits 7–8, 102
normative need 91

obsessive–compulsive disorder 60,
  68
offending behaviour as outcome
  measure 43–44, 45, 50, 51, 74,
  101
opiate dependency 66
'over-inclusiveness problem' xiv

panic disorder 60, 68
paranoid personality disorder 27,
  58
parental supervision 78, 84
passive–aggressive personality
  disorder 58
paternal alcoholism 83
Personality Assessment Schedule
  (PAS) 3, 21
personality-based approach to
  psychopathy xii–xiii
personality disorders viii
  and childhood studies 75,
    81–82
  and suicide 52–53
  axis II co-occurrence 55–58, 102
  health service utilisation 88–90
  primary care studies 20–21
  problems of assessment 2–6
  problems of classification 6–9,
    102
  problems of definition 85
  problems of longitudinal
    research 43

psychobiological model 59–60
  studies in prison settings 30, 34,
    35, 38–39, 98
  studies in psychiatric settings
    24–25, 27–28
  studies in special hospitals
    39–41
Personality Disorders
  Questionnaire (PDQ) 14, 17, 56
phobic disorder 60, 68
primary care studies 20–24, 100
prison settings, studies in 28–39,
  67, 92, 98, 100
protective factors 84, 100, 101
psychiatric settings, studies in
  24–28, 100
psychiatric syndromes,
  co-occurrence with 2–3, 58–68
psychobiological model of
  personality disorders 59–60
psychopathic disorder as legal
  category xi, 40, 41–42, 45, 101
psychopathic inferiorities x
psychopathic personalities x
psychopathy
  and criminality 34, 88
  and substance misuse 67
  as clinical construct xi–xv
  as legal category xi, 40, 41–42,
    45, 101
  behaviour-based approach
    xiii–xv
  Blackburn's model 8–9
  concept and relationship to
    antisocial personality disorder
    ix, x–xv, xvi, 100, 101–102
  fledgling psychopaths 77
  needs assessment 96–99
  personality-based approach
    xii–xiii
  treatability 98–99
Psychopathy Checklist (PCL) xi,
  xii, 33, 51, 88
Psychopathy Checklist, revised
  (PCL–R) xii, xv
psychosexual dysfunction 60

psychosocial outcome variables,
  need for 101
psychotic disorder 61

racial differences 20
reconviction as outcome measure
  43–44, 45, 51, 101
Reed Report 1994 viii, 96, 101
remand population studies 35–39, 92
risk factor studies 2, 70–84, 101
  childhood antecedents 74–84
  genetic studies 70–74, 77

sampling decisions 15–16
Schedule for Affective Disorders
  and Schizophrenia (Lifetime
  Version) (SADS–L) 14, 17–18
schizophrenia 25, 60, 68
Schneider's 10 pathological
  personality types x, 6
second-generation studies 11
selection/referral bias 10–11
self-report questionnaires,
  problems of 3, 6, 9, 56
sentenced population studies 30–35
severity criterion 95
sex offenders 8, 88
sexual abuse 81
social and health care burden
  studies 2, 85–90, 93
sociocultural biases 3
socio-economic status 19, 79
sociopathy ix, xiv, xvi, 27–28, 40, 44
somatisation disorder 24, 72
special/high security hospitals,
  studies in 39–42
Special Hospitals Assessment of
  Personality and Socialisation 9

Standardised Assessment of
  Personality (SAP) 3
state effects 59, 66
Structured Interview for
  Personality Disorders (SIDP) 14
substance misuse xiv, 33, 60, 61,
  62–67, 68, 86, 89, 98
suicide 52–54, 60, 86
symptoms, frequency of 20

Taiwan 17
temperament in childhood,
  studies of 79–81
third-generation studies 11–12
tobacco use disorder 60
traumatic childhood experiences
  81–84
treatability issue 98–99, 101
treatment needs of mentally
  disordered offenders 34, 38–39,
  40–41, 98–99
twin studies 71–72

undercontrolled temperament 80,
  81, 101
'under-inclusiveness problem' xiv
unemployment 86
unnatural deaths 54
urban/rural differences 19

victimisation in childhood 82–83
violent crime 81, 83, 86–88

wife battering 86
women 3, 18, 34–35, 38, 39

young people, needs assessment
  for 97–98